The Psychiatric Consult

Alyson Gorun
Anna M. Kim
Christian Umfrid
Janna Gordon-Elliot
Editors

The Psychiatric Consult

Navigating Challenging Treatment Plans

Second Edition

Springer

Editors
Alyson Gorun
Weill Cornell Medicine
New York-Presbyterian Hospital
New York, NY, USA

Anna M. Kim
Icahn School of Medicine at
Mount Sinai
New York, NY, USA

Christian Umfrid
Weill Cornell Medicine
New York-Presbyterian Hospital
New York, NY, USA

Janna Gordon-Elliot
Weill Cornell Medicine
New York-Presbyterian Hospital
New York, NY, USA

ISBN 978-3-031-26836-6 ISBN 978-3-031-26837-3 (eBook)
https://doi.org/10.1007/978-3-031-26837-3

This Springer imprint is published by the registered company Springer Nature Switzerland AG
The registered company address is: Gewerbestrasse 11, 6330 Cham, Switzerland

Paper in this product is recyclable

Contents

Contributors

Jonathan Avery Department of Psychiatry, NewYork-Presbyterian Hospital, New York, NY, USA

Melanie Bilbul Department of Psychiatry and Addictology, University of Montreal, Montreal, QC, Canada

Anne Clark-Raymond NewYork-Presbyterian Hospital/Weill Cornell Medicine, New York, NY, USA

Ariella R. Dagi Department of Psychiatry, NewYork-Presbyterian Hospital/Weill Cornell Medicine, New York, NY, USA

Jessica Daniels Adult Outpatient Behavioral Health, Baystate Medical Center, Springfield, MA, USA

Anna Dickerman Department of Psychiatry, NewYork-Presbyterian Hospital/Weill Cornell Medicine, New York, NY, USA

Carrie Ernst Department of Psychiatry, Icahn School of Medicine at Mount Sinai, New York, NY, USA

Department of Medical Education, Icahn School of Medicine at Mount Sinai, New York, NY, USA

Jennifer Finkel Department of Psychiatry, Icahn School of Medicine at Mount Sinai, New York, NY, USA

Liliya Gershengoren New York University Medical Center, New York, NY, USA

Janna Gordon-Elliot Weill Cornell Medicine, New York-Presbyterian Hospital, New York, NY, USA

Alyson Gorun Weill Cornell Medicine, New York-Presbyterian Hospital, New York, NY, USA

Alison Hermann Department of Psychiatry, NewYork-Presbyterian Hospital/Weill Cornell Medicine, New York, NY, USA

Kristopher A. Kast Department of Psychiatry and Behavioral Sciences, Vanderbilt University Medical Center, Nashville, TN, USA

Anna M. Kim Icahn School of Medicine at Mount Sinai, New York, NY, USA

Rachel Knight Department of Psychiatry, NewYork-Presbyterian Hospital/Weill Cornell Medicine, New York, NY, USA

Omar Mirza Department of Psychiatry, Harlem Hospital, New York, NY, USA

Chloe Nims Department of Psychiatry, NewYork-Presbyterian Hospital/Weill Cornell Medicine, New York, NY, USA

Julie Penzner Department of Psychiatry, Duke Regional Hospital, Durham, NC, USA

Jasdeep Sandhu Department of Psychiatry, Dell Medical School- The University of Texas at Austin, Austin, TX, USA

Christina Shayevitz Department of Psychiatry, NewYork-Presbyterian Hospital/Weill Cornell Medicine, New York, NY, USA

Jessica Spellun Department of Psychiatry, NewYork-Presbyterian Hospital/Weill Cornell Medicine, New York, NY, USA

Christian Umfrid Weill Cornell Medicine, New York-Presbyterian Hospital, New York, NY, USA

Introduction

1

Alyson Gorun, Christian Umfrid, and Janna Gordon-Elliot

As reported by Lavakumar et al. [1], when clinicians from seven different academic centers across the United States were asked to rate what factors were most important to them when requesting a psychiatric consultation, two of the three most important parameters identified were "understanding the core questions being asked" and "practical and helpful management suggestions for medical staff". Understanding the consult question and providing actionable recommendations are not as straightforward tasks as they may first seem. The consult question may be incomplete, misleading, or not easily discernible. It may be prompted by a number of different needs or tensions, some of them practical (e.g., "the patient is not taking his medications"), or interpersonal (e.g., dynamic processes between the patient and the team, between the patient's illness and the team, or among team members). The *ask*, or help, that the consultee is requesting may indeed be "practical" (e.g., "what medication will help manage this behavior?") or more intangible (e.g., a wish for the patient to be cured of an untreatable illness, or a desire that the patient not be

A. Gorun (✉) · C. Umfrid · J. Gordon-Elliot
Weill Cornell Medicine, New York-Presbyterian Hospital, New York, NY, USA
e-mail: jsg2005@med.cornell.edu

A. Gorun et al. (eds.), *The Psychiatric Consult*,
https://doi.org/10.1007/978-3-031-26837-3_1

the team's "problem" any longer). Sometimes the physician requesting the consult cannot quite articulate what the exact issue is, or what kind of help they are requesting—only that there is *something* impeding the course of treatment and that assistance is needed to bring the situation back into usual order. While it can be relatively straightforward—although never simple—to learn the basics of how to manage common clinical problems and patient presentations seen on the Consultation-Liaison (C-L) Psychiatry service, it is substantially more challenging to gain proficiency in handling the many layers that lie beneath the surface of the typical consult, from psychodynamic complexity to the external influences of the medical system. This book aims to fill that gap and provide insight into the parts of the consultation process that require the consultation-liaison psychiatrist to think beyond the facts of the consult.

This case-based book is written from the trainee perspective in order to create a realistic and real-time experience of what it is like to complete a psychiatric consultation. Unlike many other texts, these cases aim to help you to integrate all of the data available to you as a psychiatrist, including how you *feel* with a patient or with other members of the medical team. Attunement to this and other aspects of the complicated dynamics that occur within a medical system, between patients and clinicians, and amongst medical team members, is often times the crucial missing component to gaining a better understanding of the patient or the challenges faced by the primary team, as well as effectively answering the primary team's consult question.

Each chapter within this book will start with a message from the consulting primary team. These consult requests will often be vague, or unintentionally misleading, similar to a real consult question you might receive while working on the C-L psychiatry service. Various potential interpretations of that pager message will be outlined, followed by a description of the process of gathering key information about the patient, and the initial conversation between the C-L psychiatry trainee who received the consult request and the medical resident who requested the consult. Next, the chapter will discuss three different clinical scenarios stemming from that initial vignette, walking you step-by-step through the process of deconstructing the consult. This will include descriptions of further discussions with the primary team, interactions with the patient and family members, and the approach to formulating an assessment of the patient and recommendations for the primary team. In parallel with these descriptions, clues pointing to underlying psychodynamic factors are described. Each chapter and clinical scenario is anchored in a psychiatric diagnosis or key concept, but like most consults, will veer into unexpected areas as the case unfolds. At the conclusion of each chapter, a practical summary table of problems and strategies are listed, offering clinical pearls regarding addressing patient symptoms and behaviors, provider-patient dynamics, inter-provider and provider-family dynamics, patient-provider barriers, and hospital system barriers.

We hope this book helps you as a member of the C-L team learn how to approach the psychiatric consult from a new perspective, and how to enjoy it!

Reference

1. Lavakumar M, Gastelum ED, Choo T-H, Gerkin JS, Kahn D, Lee S, et al. Parameters of consultee satisfaction with inpatient academic psychiatric consultation services: a multicenter study. Psychosomatics. 2015;56(3):262–7.

Delirium

2

Alyson Gorun, Anna M. Kim,
and Janna Gordon-Elliot

Your pager reads: "I think he's confused"

This page is a statement, but—fundamentally—it's a question. The first question you can ask the consult requestor is: How is the patient "confused?" With this question, you are starting the process of teasing out which element of the mental status exam or overall presentation the primary team is concerned about; specifically, you are clarifying whether there is a problem with cognition and awareness. If the response indicates that confusion is present, then what kind of confusion? In other words, what are the core elements of the presentation, and what might be the etiology of the confusion? The primary team's assessment of "confusion" may also refer to a behavior, such as agitation, in which case recommendations about managing problematic behavior may be part of this consult. They may also be wondering, or wanting to know, whether the "confusion" is related to a psychiatric condition, or

A. Gorun (✉) · J. Gordon-Elliot
Weill Cornell Medicine, New York-Presbyterian Hospital,
New York, NY, USA
e-mail: jsg2005@med.cornell.edu

A. M. Kim
Icahn School of Medicine at Mount Sinai, New York, NY, USA
e-mail: akim19@northwell.edu

A. Gorun et al. (eds.), *The Psychiatric Consult*,
https://doi.org/10.1007/978-3-031-26837-3_2

whether this is the reason the patient is not adherent with treatment, and—if so—how to make the patient easier to care for safely and effectively.

Clinical Scenario

You take a look at the chart and call the primary team back. When the medical resident on the phone tells you about the patient, he seems distracted and uninterested. He says that this patient came in after being found on the street by police. The patient was confused about where he was and was unable to provide a coherent history, so he doesn't have a lot of information to tell you. He doesn't even know what his name is and thinks he might have another chart in the electronic medical record somewhere he can't find. When you start asking more clarifying questions the resident stops you and says he really doesn't have any other information and instead mentions all of the other medically sick patients he has right now on the floor. He adds that he has to go in a minute to take care of them.

Scenario 1: Delirium

On the chart review you conducted before you called the medical resident back, you discovered that the patient received multiple doses of haloperidol and lorazepam overnight. You ask what behaviors the patient exhibited overnight that led to the medications being given, and the resident says that he heard from the overnight team that the patient was cursing at staff loudly and throwing things at them when they tried to draw blood or insert an intravenous line, which is very different from how he presents when the day team evaluates him. During the day, the patient is mostly asleep which prevents them from obtaining further history from him. The primary team is placing the consult today because the overnight staff from the entire floor have complained that they can't control his agitation. The resident on the phone sounds annoyed and says he doesn't have time to keep him "in check" and wants recommendations for medications to help him be more "compliant"—otherwise how can they help him medically? You notice what you believe to be the team's feeling of frustration toward the patient as a result of their conceptualizing the patient as intentionally thwarting treatment, when (you suspect) he likely has an altered mental status. They're asking some of the right questions, you think to yourself: they are calling the patient "confused," which, indeed, he appears to be, and they are asking for help managing him, which you can offer. Nonetheless, what appears to be an essential element of this consult—and something you as the psychiatric consultant will want to help with in some way—is the team and staff's misinterpretation of the patient's behavior and subsequent over-medication, and the emotional responses they appear to be having to the patient's presentation.

With your initial hypothesis formulated, you go to see the patient. It is still morning and he's asleep. You try to wake him up by introducing yourself loudly but he doesn't respond, and then try to tap his shoulder but he swats you away. You experience your own sense of frustration at the patient and inability to engage in an interview—now you'll have to come back later and you will end up spending more time on this patient than you had initially allotted. You probably won't have the information you need before you see your attending on rounds, you think to yourself, and you worry about the attending's impression of your competence. You then realize that this response, itself, is information! You wonder if these are some of the thoughts and feelings that the team is experiencing and reacting to.

In the late afternoon when you try to interview the patient again you find that he is more alert. The patient immediately asks you a question that hints at his disorientation, and when you ask him where he is, he names a homeless shelter nearby the hospital. You ask him if there's anyone that he knows that you can call to get more information, and he tells you the name of a pastor and the name of the church he goes to. You are able to ask a couple of more questions to assess his level of orientation before he becomes increasingly irritable and asks you to leave. You ask one final question before leaving about whether he is suicidal or homicidal, and he emphatically shouts "no!" You call the pastor after finding his name on the internet and not only are you able to find the patient's name, Mr. L, but also learn from the pastor that this patient has been going to church every week prior to this hospitalization and that the pastor knows him quite well. At his baseline, he is not confused or irritable and in fact was cognitively intact enough to help him organize church outings as recently as a few weeks ago. The pastor had been worried about him since he hadn't seen him last Sunday, and appreciated the call.

You go back to the primary team to discuss your diagnostic impression and recommendations. Given the acute onset of disorientation and fluctuating presentation of his symptoms, your most likely diagnosis at this point is delirium. You suspect that the medications for agitation he receives at night likely leads to him being sedated all day, which perpetuates a disrupted sleep/wake cycle. You validate the team's frustration regarding this challenging patient and how difficult it is to manage complaints from staff about a patient that gets agitated overnight when they are not on call. You provide psychoeducation about delirium, including standard delirium precautions (Table 2.1). Regarding the behavior overnight, you give medication recommendations for agitation, and emphasize that it will be important for the day team to clearly communicate the protocol to the night team—including clear

Table 2.1 Precautions for reducing delirium in the hospital setting [1–3]

- Reorient the patient frequently
- Provide environmental orientation cues (e.g., visible clock, calendar/date, family photos, familiar objects)
- Address sensory impairments (e.g., hearing aids, eyeglasses)
- Move patient to window bed for day/night orientation
- Minimize disruptions to sleep/wake cycle by clustering care to daytime, maintaining daytime wakefulness, reducing alarms and noncritical interventions overnight
- Encourage early mobility
- Minimize use of unnecessary lines and tethers (e.g., IV lines, telemetry leads, restraints)
- Minimize use of deliriogenic medications (e.g., benzodiazepines, opioids, corticosteroids, drugs with anticholinergic and antihistaminergic activity)

indications to give medications for agitation with an overarching goal to minimize their use in order to allow the patient to be alert during the day.

Discussing the etiology of Mr. L's behavior with the primary team can help them reframe their meaning—no longer is this a patient who is purposely interfering with care, but a medically ill and disoriented patient who has little control over his actions. By providing the team with clear recommendations on how to manage his behavioral dysregulation overnight, you are directly addressing their consult question, as well as offering them means to feel more in control of the situation.

In this scenario, the staff and residents feel out of control and the floor may even feel afraid of this agitated patient, but the day team only sees an overmedicated and sleeping patient. The discrepancy in assessments between the day and night teams helps support your diagnosis of delirium. You theorize that the patient's dysregulated pattern of arousal due to the delirium contributed to problematic behavior at night, leading to his receiving excessive medications, in turn preventing a correction of sleep-wake cycle and his altered mental status. All of these affect discharge planning. Obtaining collateral allows you to not only clarify the diagnosis but also to help you humanize the patient for yourself and for the team. Addressing what is behind the team's frustration can often be informed by using your own countertransference as a clue. Your own sense of frustration at the patient is likely similar to what the team is feeling. Further reflection allows you to see how even your assessment of the overnight treatment as "overmedicating," and the annoyance you found yourself feeling at the night team for this "mistake," is a countertransference signal. You are finding yourself vacillating between being frustrated at the team and protective of the patient, to feeling frustrated at the whole situation (e.g., the disregard you are picking up from the consulting resident, the time this consult is taking, etc.) and throwing your hands up in the air. These and other reactions can be discussed within your psychiatry team. This can then be used to empathize with the overworked medicine residents and staff while also providing guidance to help the patient in a meaningful way.

Scenario 2: Hypoactive Delirium

While on the phone with the primary team during your initial callback, a medical student they had sent to interview the patient returns and says they were able to find out the patient's name and date of birth. The medical resident says they'll call you back after they review Mr. L's chart now that they have his identifying information. The next day, you get a phone call from the same resident saying that they were able to get more information—Mr. L had been diagnosed with colon cancer a couple of years ago and now has metastases to his brain. The resident says that he understands that the behavior at night is related to acute mental status changes, and they've implemented a behavioral and treatment plan for overnight management, but now they are calling you because they wonder whether Mr. L is also depressed. He doesn't respond to any of their questions, has a lack of energy, and isn't eating. They also say the social worker has tried multiple times to discuss with him different disposition options for when he leaves the hospital but Mr. L only responds with the word "home." When they try to talk to him about his cancer diagnosis he is disengaged and responds in one word answers if at all. They don't know how else to convey details of his diagnosis and treatment and aren't sure if he is being stubborn, is "in denial" about his illness, is depressed, or something else.

When you enter the room of Mr. L later in the afternoon, the patient looks nothing like what you were expecting based on the medical resident's description. The room is full of people speaking a language you've never heard. The visitors have brought food from home and Mr. L is eating. Mr. L is also responding readily to their questions. You confirm that this is Mr. L's family and you find out that he speaks an unusual dialect of a rare language and that not every interpreter would necessarily understand. When you call the interpreter to speak to Mr. L, you confirm he is speaking that specific dialect. Although he has some difficulty on many domains of the mental status exam, especially in the domains measuring attention, he was engaged with the interview. He told you he only wants to eat food that is cooked from home, and understands that he may not be able to go home because he has been having difficulty taking care of himself at home due to his medical condition. The family also confirms there has been a slow decline in his cognitive status, but that his getting lost on the street concerned and scared them since this was a sudden change from his baseline.

When you get back on the phone with the primary team you share with them your impressions that he likely has a neurocognitive disorder with a superimposed hypoactive delirium, given his fluctuating symptoms (e.g., the discrepant presentation between the primary team's description and when you interviewed Mr. L), inattentive symptoms on his mental status exam, and recent acute decline as reported by his family. They are surprised to hear that Mr. L was eating and engaging with his family. You ask them if they've been using an interpreter phone and also know about this specific dialect—and they replied they used it "as much as we could" but thought he was able to understand enough without using it. The resident goes on to say—"I just don't know what to do with these patients... I don't feel like there's anything I can do to make them better."

You wonder if the team feels ineffective, helpless and defeated, and may be avoiding spending the time with an interpreter phone or engaging with the family because they believe it will have little effect. Perhaps the team feels demoralized that they are unable to help this end-stage cancer patient, or that "they" (the medical system) weren't able to prevent the spread of his cancer; such experiences, especially if not in conscious awareness, can shake the confidence of physicians, as it calls into question, on some level, their capacity to help, fix, and cure. Physicians in training may be particularly susceptible to such feelings, as so much of their work at this point is mastering the knowledge and skills needed to diagnose and treat disease; factors that interfere with, or otherwise alter, these algorithms, can be destabilizing. Sharing an interpretation like this with the team is usually not the best option; though aspects of it can be expressed in small ways (e.g., by validating how hard it is to see a potentially curable disease progress). Rather than interpreting what is happening, you can turn your attention to supporting and empowering the team in their care of the patient. You can frame your recommendations as active interventions, such as finding appropriate placement for the patient, or utilizing palliative care or other consults to alleviate the patient's symptoms. Sometimes just letting teams know of different options or approaches that fulfill their desire to "do something" or "fix something" can lead to better engagement. You can share the information that you discovered about the patient's primary language, and gently suggest attempting to use the interpreter phone for all communications. It might add to the length of the interview, you say, but it could further help engage and understand what is actually happening so as to make a realistic plan for care and discharge, thus ultimately moving things along more effectively. Additionally, the help of family could provide a more fruitful discussion of the disposition plan to be attained. You can explain that appropriate communication and coordination of care are both key here to optimize care and prevent a hospital bounce-back. Being unaware of cultural factors and a patient's level of health literacy can affect the therapeutic alliance and impact treatment and thus should always be kept at the forefront of your mind.

Scenario 3: Neurocognitive Disorder

The primary team calls you back a short while after the initial consult phone call and says that the patient's daughter arrived at the hospital and gave them the patient's name—and now the team can see his prior medical record. The primary team has concluded that the patient's presentation is from his underlying neurocognitive disorder, but his daughter disagrees and says that there is an active medical issue that must be treated. You take a quick look at Mr. L's chart and don't see any of the common factors contributing to delirium other than advanced age (see Table 2.2 for a brief list of risk factors for delirium). Nothing stands out in the chart: he has no chronic illnesses, his laboratory values are within normal limits, there are no recent surgeries, and he's not receiving any deliriogenic medications. The medical resident on the phone says that the family member, Mr. L's daughter, is saying that her father is completely off his baseline and is irritated that the primary team has not given a diagnosis other than a neurocognitive disorder. The daughter says that her father lives alone at home and typically is easily able to take care of himself and the whole family. Now she has concerns he can no longer do so and wants the primary team to treat him so that he can return to his baseline.

Table 2.2 Common risk factors for delirium [2–4]

- Advanced age
- Neurocognitive disorders
- Other disorders and injuries to the brain, including hypoperfusion
- Severe medical illness
- Infectious illness
- Traumatic injuries, including burns and orthopedic injuries
- Deliriogenic medication burden and polypharmacy
- Metabolic and electrolyte derangements
- Drug and alcohol intoxication or withdrawal
- Sensory impairments
- Hospital environment, including circadian rhythm disruptions

The resident asks you whether there could be a psychiatric contribution to Mr. L's presentation that could be treated, and if you could see him to rule this out.

When you go to see Mr. L he is awake and alert and greets you politely. You introduce yourself and your role, and he smiles and says, "I don't need a psychiatrist, but they all do!", pointing outside his door to the empty hallway. His daughter is at his bedside. You introduce yourself and try to ask orientation questions. He laughs and fumbles with the answers, all the while you notice the daughter quickly jump in to answer for him. She reminds him of the details of his hospital course and treatment before he has time to answer your questions. You also notice yourself enjoying Mr. L's jokes and gently guiding him in answering your questions to not make him uncomfortable. You find out that she only communicates with him via phone once a week and lives across the country with her husband and children. Additionally, Mr. L's wife passed away about a year ago.

You decide to review his chart more in depth including looking at records outside his current inpatient hospitalization. You see that Mr. L has a primary care provider, who is at your institution. You uncover a Montreal Cognitive Assessment (MoCA) exam documented at a recent office visit of 25/30. The note also mentions that the doctor is concerned about his increasing forgetfulness and difficulty completing his basic activities of daily living (ADLs). You reflect on Mr. L's jocular but superficial way of expressing himself during your visit, consistent with confabulation due to declining cognitive function. He did appear mildly disheveled, too, but you notice how you minimized this, and you wonder if the presence of the competent daughter in the room made you overlook that.

You wonder if this is actually Mr. L's baseline. Does he have a neurocognitive disorder that the patient's daughter does not want to be aware of? When you go back to the daughter and you mention the concern for forgetfulness by the primary care doctor, she then recalls that he had called her a couple of times in the past few months not sure where he was. These calls were made by him well after midnight, but because of their 3 hour time difference, she realizes that she hadn't made note of how late that was for him. He also sometimes called her by his wife's name, which she has laughed off as a simple mistake. When you suggest that perhaps his current presentation is part of a slow cognitive decline, she becomes defensive and says that she knows her father and this isn't him—something medically needs to be done now. You wonder if her demand may be related to a difficulty in processing his diagnosis. When you ask her about herself a bit more, you hear about a number of stressors both at home and at work, and validate how overwhelmed she feels. She feels guilty about not being there more for her father given all of her responsibilities to her children and husband and job, and wonders that maybe she didn't quite recognize her father's declining condition.

It appears that the daughter may now be more able to acknowledge her father's diagnosis and treatment recommendations from the team. Denial, anger, sadness, guilt, as well as other emotions can be common responses to changes in the health or functional status of a family member. In this case, you suspect that the daughter's complicated emotions related to her emerging, but unwanted, realization of her father's cognitive decline, is manifesting in interpersonal friction between her and the team, and a request for help from the primary team in the form of a psychiatric consult. By recognizing and validating such reactions, the psychiatric consultant can actually begin to lay the ground for a more realistic understanding and a more open dialogue. As a result, the work of the admission can progress—from diagnosis, to management, to aftercare planning, making for a more effective, and meaningful, clinical experience for everyone.

Appendix: Summary Table

	Problems	Strategies
• Patient symptoms and behaviors	• Cognitive: Confusion, disorientation, inattention • Psychosis: Paranoia and suspiciousness of staff resulting in fear, refusal of workup and treatment • Behavioral disturbances: Agitation, combativeness, affective lability	• Assist with diagnostic clarification and support the team in identifying and addressing underlying etiology of delirium • Provide guidance in minimizing iatrogenic and environmental contributions to delirium (Table 2.1) • Offer easy-to-follow management recommendations, including behavioral strategies for patient redirection, reorientation, and reassurance, active engagement • Consider pharmacologic interventions for managing agitation and distressing psychotic symptoms that are interfering with safety or treatment. May also aid in directing team's approach to agitation and reducing use of restraints and polypharmacy
• Provider-patient dynamics	• Provider has feelings of demoralization and ineffectiveness in their care. May mobilize defensive sense of boredom and disengagement, anger, and frustration, or be projected onto patient as distress or emergence of "depression" • Patient agitation and irritability is contributing to staff fearfulness, sense of disempowerment and lack of control, avoidance, over-medicating	• Provide a clear diagnosis and psychoeducation, help the team recognize signs of delirium, make sense of frustrating or frightening behaviors, and reengage them in medical workup and management • Outline active interventions to be made to help the patient and re-empower the team • Validate and empathize with team frustrations and concerns while supporting their continued thoughtful care for the patient

	Problems	Strategies
• Inter-provider and provider-family dynamics	• Team attributes symptoms to an underlying psychiatric disorder (e.g. depression, psychotic disorder), leading to sense of being de-skilled, loss of "ownership" of treatment, a drive to transfer patient, or limiting further medical management • Family distressed about acute cognitive and behavioral changes, or medical and physical interventions being used for management	• Provide a clear diagnosis and psychoeducation for the primary team and family. May remark explicitly if there are no primary psychiatric comorbidities or contributions to current presentation • Assist in guiding and expanding primary team's thinking about the etiology further workup of the delirium to reengage • Consider continuing to follow and consult on the patient after evaluation to collaborate and provide team with support • Educate family about delirium and expectations around recovery (if known), as well as in use of least restrictive means in effort to maintain patient's safety. Support family in their distress
• Patient-provider barriers	• English is not patient's primary language, however team or patient feels comfortable speaking without interpreter, muddying communications, and increasing mutual frustration • Cognitive impairment associated with delirium or neurocognitive disorder limiting patient's understanding in communications with providers or raising issues around capacity	• Telephonic or in-person interpreters should always be offered to patients when there is a mismatch in preferred language. Counsel and encourage primary team and patient to use interpreters to ensure complete and accurate communication, and that all parties feel heard • Provide cognitively impaired patients with clear, simple, and concrete explanations. Identify and elicit support from family or next of kin

	Problems	Strategies
• Hospital system barriers	• Patient requires higher level of care upon discharge from hospital, however no facilities will accept them due to recurrent agitation, need for direct observation for wandering or falls, or use of restraints	• Consider additional provider and staff education around behavioral management and redirection, standing pharmacologic interventions for frequent agitation, and creative changes in environment to make use of least restrictive means necessary for safety (e.g., bed placement, bed and unit alarms for wandering)

References

1. Inouye SK, Bogardus ST Jr, Charpentier PA, Leo-Summers L, Acampora D, Holford TR, Cooney LM Jr. A multicomponent intervention to prevent delirium in hospitalized older patients. N Engl J Med. 1999;4:669–76.
2. Inouye SK, Westendorp RGJ, Saczynski JS. Delirium in elderly people. Lancet. 2014;383:911–22.
3. Leentjens AFG, Meagher DJ. Delirium. In: Levenson J, editor. The American Psychiatric Association Publishing textbook of psychosomatic medicine and consultation-liaison psychiatry. 3rd ed. Washington, DC: American Psychiatric Association; 2019.
4. Caplan JP. Delirious patients. In: Stern TA, Freudenreich O, Smith FA, Fricchione GL, Rosenbaum JF, editors. Massachusetts General Hospital handbook of general hospital psychiatry. 7th ed. Amsterdam: Elsevier; 2018.

Further Reading

Levenson JL, Ferrando SF, editors. Clinical manual of psychopharmacology in the medically ill. 2nd ed. Arlington: American Psychiatry Association; 2017.

Altered Mental Status

3

Christian Umfrid
and Liliya Gershengoren

The pager reads: "The patient is still altered, could the cause be psychiatric?"

Altered mental status (AMS) is a nonspecific term used frequently in clinical settings to indicate that a patient has deviated from their baseline in behavior, level of consciousness, cognition, or in how they perceive and interact with their environment. Presentations of AMS vary widely from stuporous to agitated and combative. A change in mental status likewise can include a cluster of symptoms with a tremendously broad differential diagnosis, including toxic, metabolic and infectious etiologies, CNS pathology, psychiatric illness, and substance intoxication or withdrawal.

Psychiatric consultations for AMS are often initiated when the primary team is seeking guidance in managing behavioral disturbances, or when the team is wondering if the patient's change in mental status and behavior might be due to an underlying psychiatric disorder or its pharmacologic treatment. Once urgent behav-

C. Umfrid (✉)
Weill Cornell Medicine, New York-Presbyterian Hospital, New York, NY, USA

L. Gershengoren
New York University Medical Center, New York, NY, USA
e-mail: Liliya.gershengoren@nyulangone.org

A. Gorun et al. (eds.), *The Psychiatric Consult*,
https://doi.org/10.1007/978-3-031-26837-3_3

ioral issues are managed and safety is addressed, the team's additional concerns, such as whether underlying psychiatric issues are contributing to the patient's presentation, may remain. This is especially true—and may prompt a particularly expeditious consult request—when the patient has a known psychiatric history or presents on multiple psychotropic medications.

With this in mind, consultations involving AMS should prompt your curiosity and the question "*why consult psychiatry?*" Your initial interaction with the team allows you to begin to answer that question—what is it about the patient's history, exam or medical workup that gave rise to concerns for a possible psychiatric etiology? You might sense frustration from the primary team as a result of a lack of diagnostic clues in the workup, slow recovery with medical treatment, or around a patient's documented psychiatric diagnosis—all of which will be helpful to contextualize the consultation and clue you in to your role and how you might be most helpful. It is your task to remain diligent and unbiased in assessing the team's concerns and the patient's presentation in an effort to help clarify the diagnosis and any psychiatric contributions, to support the team and patient around concerns related to psychiatric symptoms and behavioral issues, and to ensure biases around a psychiatric diagnosis do not interfere with or unduly cloud the direction of care.

Clinical Scenario

Initial chart review reveals that the patient, Mr. K, is a 67-year-old man who has a diagnosis of schizoaffective disorder, well-documented from multiple prior psychiatric emergency room visits. He was admitted to the medicine service with "altered mental status" after being found down at home by a home health aide. The aide indicated that Mr. K had seemed to be at his cognitive and psychiatric baseline until he had begun "behaving strangely" over the week prior to admission, during which he had seemed more withdrawn and was intermittently not allowing the aide into his apartment.

After receiving the consult request, you call the primary team and the medical resident reports that the patient has been "almost nonverbal" since admission, not eating, and not interactive enough to provide any coherent history. Aside from the information obtained from the chart and aide on presentation, the team has not located other sources of collateral information. The resident states that Mr. K's head CT and infectious workup were "unremarkable," that the multiple electrolyte and metabolic derangements on presentation have corrected and do not adequately explain Mr. K's exam, and there is no remaining workup indicated. Nursing staff has expressed concern that when Mr. K does interact with them, he appears fearful, agitated, and paranoid; however the resident is not able to elaborate on these observations. The team is concerned that Mr. K remains withdrawn and altered, and question if his presentation might be "behavioral" or related to his charted diagnosis of schizoaffective disorder.

Scenario 1: Catatonia

Considering Mr. K's limited history and presentation, you begin to formulate a preliminary differential diagnosis to guide how you approach information gathering. In addition to the common causes of delirium in the medical population—many of which have increased prevalence and associated risks in patients with chronic psychiatric disorders—you consider the team's concern that there may also be decompensated mood or psychotic symptoms playing a role in his behavioral changes. You attempt to get a sense of the patient's medication adherence to inform your understanding of contributing psychiatric symptomatology, as well as risk for medication side effects, interactions, or toxicity which may be impacting Mr. K's mental status. You think of the elevated risk for suicide and substance use in patients with psychotic and affective disorders, and inquire into signs of medication overdose or toxicity, as well as signs and symptoms of recent and chronic substance use, intoxication, or withdrawal.

Altered mental status is a common cause of hospitalization, increased length of hospital stay and morbidity, but it is certainly not the case that every patient admitted with AMS requires a psychiatric consultation. You begin to ask questions of the medical resident to better understand what it is about Mr. K that has motivated the team to seek assistance from psychiatry. After the resident presents the team's concerns, you ask clarifying questions to get a better sense of Mr. K's presentation and hospital course, targeted toward understanding your role and narrowing the differential diagnosis. Mr. K's aide had told the resident that he had seemed more withdrawn, quiet, and lethargic during the week prior to presentation. On several occasions he would not answer the door or would refuse to allow the aide into his apartment. She had not seen him for 4 days before finding him unresponsive and incontinent on the floor of his apartment. She raised concern that he had not been adherent with his prescribed medications prior to these changes.

You ask about Mr. K's hospital course and exam, and the resident tells you that Mr. K has been minimally interactive, has seemed confused, has not been out of bed in 2 days, and has been "*refusing* medications and not participating in care." Upon hearing this, you wonder if there is also an underlying suspicion that some of Mr. K's behavior is volitional. You review the chart including lab results, urine toxicology screen and urinalysis, EKG, head CT, chest X-ray, and inpatient and outpatient medication lists, looking for etiologies of AMS. What stands out to you from prior psychiatric notes is that Mr. K seems to be markedly off of his documented baseline. He is also noted to be a heavy smoker, frequently medication nonadherent, and was last taking clozapine and clonazepam during a hospital presentation 4 months ago. What stands out from his workup is that he was hyponatremic on presentation, had recurrent hyponatremia when intravenous fluids were discontinued, and was found to have two suspicious pulmonary nodules on chest X-ray. Given this new information, you add to your differential diagnosis *delirium due to hyponatremia, pneumonia, lung malignancy or CNS metastases, paraneoplastic syndromes, and effects of clozapine or benzodiazepine withdrawal.*

You inquire about the findings on chest imaging and persistent sodium derangement, noting concern that they might have a role in Mr. K's presentation. The resident tells you that their team is deferring further workup to be done as an outpatient, as they have concluded that the hyponatremia is likely due to his poor nutritional intake, and the lung nodules are unrelated to his AMS. The resident tells you that he suspects Mr. K may have "unrecognized dementia" and that the team is discussing long-term disposition options following hospitalization. He asks if perhaps dementia or depression is contributing to Mr. K's apathy. He also questions if antipsychotic-related extrapyramidal symptoms might be contributing to rigidity and hypoactivity noted on Mr. K's physical exam, although it isn't clear which medications—if any—the patient has been taking.

At the end of the interaction, you're struck by the lack of clarity in Mr. K's recent history, and the vagueness in the stated goals of the consultation. You feel perplexed by the disparate neuropsychiatric concerns that have been expressed—psychosis, depression, neurocognitive disorder, apathy, medication nonadherence, extrapyramidal symptoms—and what seems to be a stalling of further investigation into Mr. K's medical issues, his life and his recent functioning outside of the hospital. You note a disconnect between the primary team discussing long-term care options for a patient they believe may have dementia, and the reality of a patient who presented with a concerning, acute (and potentially reversible) change in cognitive and functional status. You hypothesize that this may be a reflection of Mr. K's disengaged, withdrawn behavior, and the medical team's sense of confusion and feelings of helplessness given the lack of diagnosis and treatment options following his initial workup. The primary team's anxiety and inexperience with severe psychiatric disorders may motivate a tendency to identify the patient's unexplained physical and cognitive symptoms as being of a primary "psychiatric" or behavioral nature. In the setting of uncertainty about a patient's medical picture, there may be an underlying wish to attribute the unknown to a psychiatric disorder, or a hope that you as the psychiatric consultant can solve what seems like a hopeless or confounding diagnostic and treatment conundrum.

You arrive to evaluate Mr. K and find him to be stuporous, laying still in a darkened room. After opening the blinds, you scan the room for orientation cues and deliriogenic environmental factors, and observe Mr. K briefly to assess level of activity. You try repeatedly to engage him; however he appears sleepy and stares unblinking for a prolonged period of time before briefly shifting his gaze and attention to you. Mr. K responds to simple questions only intermittently and with great latency. He shuts his eyes and appears to fall asleep without continuous stimulation. You assess orientation, and Mr. K provides the incorrect year and does not respond to the remaining questions. For a moment, you find yourself sharing the feelings of hopelessness and frustration that the team may be experiencing, unable to connect with a sick patient and unable to identify a sense of certainty and direction through a clear diagnosis.

As you are not able to interview Mr. K, you readjust to relying on your mental status and neurologic exams for clues. Mr. K is rigid in all extremities, each with increasing resistance following repetitive passive movement. After examining his right arm, he holds it fixed above his body for minutes before gradually relaxing to a neutral position. You continue the exam, and Mr. K begins moaning "no...no...no..." while slowly reaching out toward you, grasping at your badge. Catatonia rises on your differential diagnosis for the patient, and you administer the Bush-Francis Catatonia Rating Scale, a validated instrument for screening and rating severity in catatonia [1]. Mr. K is withdrawn, stuporous, has a fixed gaze, is posturing and rigid, verbigerating, and demonstrating *gegenhalten*—all signs consistent with catatonia.

You begin to formulate a treatment approach, and know that first line for simple catatonia is benzodiazepines. You pause, and consider his disorientation, inattention and somnolence—while Mr. K clearly has signs of catatonia on exam, he may also have hypoactive delirium. You recognize a sense of unease with the seemingly conflicting treatment approaches for delirium and catatonia, concerned with the risk of worsening Mr. K's delirium with the addition of a benzodiazepine. You consider alternative treatment approaches—including ECT, other GABA-A receptor agonists (e.g., zolpidem), and NMDA receptor antagonists (e.g., memantine, amantadine) [2]. In your review of the literature, you note that catatonia may occur in nearly one-third of delirious patients in the medical population, and that their co-occurence contributes to the under-recognition and undertreatment of catatonia [3, 4]. Revisiting Mr. K's history and your differential provides clarity to your clinical reasoning: benzodiazepine withdrawal may be contributing to both delirium and catatonia. In fact, catatonia has a high response rate to lorazepam even in cases of comorbid delirium [5], and the medical risks associated with untreated catatonia are many and potentially severe—including decubitus ulcers, deep vein thrombosis and pulmonary embolism, aspiration, infection, dehydration, and malnutrition.

You meet with the primary team and explain your diagnostic impressions. You recommend further workup of catatonia, and explain your plan to reexamine Mr. K after a "challenge" dose of lorazepam. You describe the considerable overlap between symptoms of delirium and catatonia [2], which can often be difficult to differentiate and may co-occur, and highlight the need to monitor closely for worsening delirium as you titrate doses of benzodiazepines. The team asks if an antipsychotic should be restarted to "treat the underlying cause" of Mr. K's presentation. You use the opportunity to provide psychoeducation about the potential risk for malignant catatonia with reinitiation of an antipsychotic during an episode of catatonia You explain that Mr. K's psychopathology may have a causative role in the catatonia, but that the etiology of his current presentation remains uncertain and likely multifactorial—with the differential including benzodiazepine withdrawal, antipsychotic use or discontinuation, hyponatremia, or other undiagnosed medical or neurologic pathology. You emphasize that one-fourth to one-half of cases of catatonia may be due to general medical or neurologic processes in some populations, and is particularly concerning if it is a first episode occurring in an older adult [2, 5]. Your discussion is targeted toward broadening rather than narrowing the primary team's differential diagnosis in this case, toward activating them and re-engaging their medical curiosity in pursuit of additional workup before attributing the catatonia to an underlying psychiatric condition. You encourage the team to consider a brain MRI and EEG, further evaluation of Mr. K's pulmonary nodules and the etiology of his hyponatremia, as well as workup for nutritional and metabolic deficiencies. You note your plan to communicate with Mr. K's psychiatrist to gather more history, and to partner with the primary team in collaborative and active care of the patient. It is your role to mitigate the common pitfall of compartmentalizing the psychiatric and the medical, along with the risk for prematurely attributing symptoms to comorbid psychiatric disorders. You do so while supporting the team with diagnostic clarification, treatment collaboration, and addressing feelings of futility and disengagement that may arise along the way.

Scenario 2: Neuroleptic Malignant Syndrome and Serotonin Syndrome

The resident caring for Mr. K explains that he has been persistently "altered" since arriving to the hospital 3 days earlier, fluctuating between periods of agitation and somnolence. The team is uncertain about what might be the cause of Mr. K's altered mental status, or how best to manage his medications in the setting of an acute mental status change. After inquiring into which medications Mr. K is taking and the team's concerns, the resident tells you "he's on a lot of psychiatric medications, we aren't sure what he has actually been taking." You clarify that Mr. K is confused and unable to recall which medications he takes at home, but that his most recent charted medication list shows high doses of sertraline, lithium, and olanzapine, and there is record of many expired or discontinued antipsychotics and mood stabilizers. The resident adds that Mr. K became febrile and has been tachycardiac throughout the day, and serotonin syndrome is on the primary team's differential diagnosis. The team has already discontinued sertraline, concerned that it was contributing to his AMS; however Mr. K has remained delirious. They have repeated an infectious workup after the patient became febrile, but labs and imaging have not identified another medical etiology for his autonomic changes. The team is worried about holding all of Mr. K's psychiatric medications, as he has been agitated, appears anxious, and they are concerned about the potential for psychiatric decompensation given his well-documented history of psychosis and suicidal ideation.

You inquire about Mr. K's exam and clinical course in order to get a sense of what the resident means by "altered," and what has led to their concern for serotonin syndrome. The resident reports that Mr. K was found down at home by his aide, and has been intermittently agitated and aggressive since arriving at the hospital. Mr. K has been boarding in the emergency department for the past 3 days while awaiting a hospital room, and the nurse has paged the medical resident repeatedly to ask for medication to manage his restless and combative behavior. He had restraints placed twice overnight as staff felt unsafe caring for him. You ask about Mr. K's past medical history, and the resident adds that Mr. K has been hypertensive since admission and was rigid and tremulous on motor exam this morning, but is quick to point out his charted history of essential hypertension and neuroleptic-induced parkinsonism. You hear the resident's pager sound repeatedly over the course of the conversation, and he seems eager to end the call. The resident concludes by saying that the team "needs another set of eyes on the patient" in addition to medication guidance, noting candidly that "this is out of my wheelhouse." The resident sounds distracted and impatient with your questions, and you find yourself wondering—perhaps unfairly—if you are being asked to take over the legwork of gathering essential patient history that he does not have the time to do.

On chart review, Mr. K's medication list is indeed extensive, disorganized, and was last updated nearly 1 year ago. It contains active, expired, and discontinued medications, with numerous redundant agents from multiple drug classes. You begin to formulate an impression of Mr. K as a patient with a chronic, severe, and refractory psychotic disorder. The active medication orders and medication administration record reveal that Mr. K was initially started on sertraline and olanzapine by the admitting resident—both at their previously documented outpatient doses and that he had received multiple doses of intramuscular olanzapine and haloperidol for agitation since admission. You review the nursing notes to get a sense of the circumstances and behaviors associated with the agitation episodes, however documentation is sparse. Your initial, reactive impression that you are being consulted to help reconcile Mr. K's medication list and obtain collateral information softens to a more nuanced understanding of a primary team, overtaxed with competing demands, feeling overwhelmed and uncertain in managing a psychiatrically and medically complex patient, who is now acutely ill and unable to communicate with them. You consider your earlier experience of feeling frustrated, perplexed and anxious while speaking to the medical resident about Mr. K, and recognize that it may parallel the experience of the medical team as they work with the patient.

You find the emergency department nurse who has been caring for Mr. K for the past two nights, and she tells you that she thinks he may be manic. She describes Mr. K as somnolent and mute at present, although quite agitated on first presentation—he had been yelling out incoherently, repeating the same phrase in response to all questions, and was seen repeatedly pulling at his gown, opening nearby drawers and banging his fist on the stretcher without apparent purpose. Mr. K's nurse notes that he had also been very restless, physically intrusive, had followed her into other patients' rooms and behind the nurses' station, and had become combative whenever she redirected him. You ask about signs of serotonin syndrome, and the nurse tells you Mr. K has not had any diarrhea or vomiting, although he has been tremulous and confused. The nurse reports that the emergency department has been hectic, and she is concerned about the safety of Mr. K and the other patients when he becomes agitated. She notes that she has had to page the resident "every hour" over the past two nights to ask for more medication when the patient seems restless and begins to escalate behaviorally. Mr. K has been more sedated since receiving medication earlier that morning, although is still confused and swatting at her when she attempts to provide hands-on care. While gathering more details about his behavior and response to medication, the nurse interjects to ask "when are you going to transfer him to psychiatry? He's too agitated to stay here." With this question you sense that, like the medical resident, she may also be communicating that she feels overwhelmed, fearful, and *stuck* in taking care of Mr. K, who has been impulsive, disorganized, and intermittently aggressive. You express understanding and empathize with the fear, frustration and anger that can accompany caring for a combative and unpredictable patient, knowing that it can be helpful to name and validate these uncomfortable thoughts and feelings. In the process, you hope to also begin to reduce the risk of Mr. K's providers unintentionally acting in response to their anxiety with avoidance of the patient or use of unnecessary physical and pharmacological interventions.

You see Mr. K and he is laying askew in bed, his legs overhanging the side rail. He appears mildly diaphoretic, restless and writhing, and does not respond as you try to engage him. You reposition his legs back into the bed and note marked resistance in doing so. He is severely and diffusely rigid in all extremities, with subtle cogwheel rigidity in his upper extremities bilaterally. Mr. K is able to follow some commands with repeat prompting and encouragement, and you see that his arms are tremulous as he slowly extends them. Mr. K's reflexes are diminished, and you do not elicit clonus. You review his monitor and see that he remains hypertensive and tachycardiac in absence of agitation. As you leave the emergency room, you ask the nurse to hold all antipsychotic medications until you are able to discuss your impression and treatment options with the primary team. She agrees, however appears distressed and presses for recommendations on what to do if Mr. K becomes agitated again. You wonder if Mr. K may have been overmedicated, the high dosing of multiple neuroleptics, and the resumption of lithium and the selective serotonin reuptake inhibitor overlooked or decided in haste by an overwhelmed treatment team, perhaps unduly influenced by fear of Mr. K's behavior and concerns about his psychiatric history. You offer your assessment of the patient's behavior, and assure the nurse you will provide her with a clear plan for safely managing his agitation in the emergency room.

Mr. K's differential diagnosis remains broad, but considering the fluctuations in his mental status and level of consciousness, his motor exam, and the progression of his symptoms in relationship to medication changes, both serotonin syndrome and neuroleptic malignant syndrome (NMS) are of highest concern. You reflect on Mr. K's exam and vital sign changes and are unable to clearly differentiate between NMS and serotonin syndrome, knowing that there is considerable overlap in the symptoms of each condition. Both commonly share autonomic instability, altered mental status, and agitation. You consider their distinguishing features hoping to find diagnostic clarity, recalling that serotonin syndrome is associated with more gastrointestinal symptoms, hyperreflexia, and myoclonus, while NMS is associated with rigidity, hyporeflexia, and rhabdomyolysis (Table 3.1) [6]. You consider lab tests which may provide further evidence to identify a diagnosis of NMS. While the exam findings associated with each syndrome are descriptively unique, you recognize that both can present with a range of symptoms and severity, and try to correlate Mr. K's symptom onset with his medication changes and supportive lab values.

Collateral information is critical to understanding Mr. K's presentation and formulating a plan, so you begin by clarifying his medical and psychiatric history, as well as information obtained from his aide. You learn that Mr. K was managing medications himself, and had not seen a psychiatrist or refilled his antipsychotic medication in many months. In reviewing documentation from prior psychiatric hospitalizations, you find that the inpatient psychiatric team had previously suspected Mr. K to have excited catatonia, which had presented with restless, agitated, and combative behavior, symptoms that were also initially misattributed to mania. Excited catatonia rises on your differential diagnosis for Mr. K's initial presentation, given the description of psychomotor agitation, impulsivity, motor stereotypies, perseveration and echophenomena. You hypothesize that Mr. K may be catatonic, and that high doses of multiple antipsychotics which had been rapidly escalated may have precipitated NMS, a specific subtype of malignant catatonia [7]. Mr. K's risk for NMS may have been further increased by dehydration, agitation, antidepressant or lithium administration, as well as excited catatonia itself [8, 9].

Review of the chart also reveals that olanzapine was initiated at a high dose immediately on admission, and multiple doses of haloperidol were administered soon thereafter, while Mr. K was unable to provide the history that he had not been taking these medications prior to hospitalization. You think about the overex-

Table 3.1 Common and differentiating features of serotonin syndrome and neuroleptic malignant syndrome [6]

	Serotonin syndrome	Neuroleptic malignant syndrome
• Etiology	• Serotonergic antidepressants • Triptans • Meperidine • Tramadol • Linezolid • Methylenedioxymethamphetamine (MDMA)	• Antipsychotic drugs (typical or atypical) • Rapid discontinuation of dopamine agonists • Antiemetic drugs
• Autonomic signs	• Fever • Tachycardia • Hypertension	• Fever • Tachycardia • Hypertension
• Exam findings	• Altered mental status • Agitation • Clonus • Tremor • Hyperreflexia • Rigidity • Mydriasis • Diaphoresis	• Altered mental status • Agitation • No clonus • Tremor • Hyporeflexia • Rigidity (severe or “lead pipe”) • No pupillary changes • Diaphoresis
• Symptoms	• Nausea, vomiting, diarrhea • Rhabdomyolysis	• No gastrointestinal symptoms • Rhabdomyolysis

(continued)

Table 3.1 (continued)

	Serotonin syndrome		Neuroleptic malignant syndrome
• Labs	• Leukocytosis • Creatine kinase (elevated) • Myoglobinuria		• Leukocytosis • Creatine kinase (highly elevated) • Myoglobinuria • Proteinuria • Lactate dehydrogenase (elevated) • AST/ALT (elevated) • Serum iron levels (low)

tended resident and nurse caring for Mr. K, and consider if feelings of inexperience with psychiatric management, misperceptions about the unpredictability of aggression in patients with psychiatric disorders, misattributions of patient intent and volitionality in his agitation, and worries about the fragility of the most feared psychiatric symptoms (e.g., suicidality and psychosis) may have contributed to reactive medication initiation prior to confirming adherence, and aggressive antipsychotic dosing. When you call the resident to provide recommendations—which include discontinuing and avoiding use of all dopamine antagonists, continuing to hold lithium and sertraline, managing agitation and catatonia with benzodiazepines, and considering initial treatment with dantrolene, and/or bromocriptine along with supportive care—you also provide education about your diagnostic impression. You emphasize that the consult service will follow closely to support the team in managing Mr. K's neuropsychiatric symptoms. In clearly identifying the reasons for Mr. K's combative behavior, explicitly supporting the urgent discontinuation of antipsychotic medications, and emphasizing your plan for continued involvement in his psychiatric management, you aim to reduce the team's anxiety, reduce psychiatric misperceptions and unspoken fear, and provide safe and collaborative care for the patient as he is treated in the hospital.

Scenario 3: Wernicke Encephalopathy

After hearing from the primary team that Mr. K is admitted with AMS and cannot provide accurate history, you turn to a close review of his medical and psychiatric chart to inform your assessment and target your interview and exam to your differential diagnosis. Chart review reveals that Mr. K has been confused and disoriented since he presented to the emergency department 4 days ago. He was lethargic on arrival, now improved with supportive care, but is noted to have a waxing and waning level of alertness. Nursing notes provide an initial impression of Mr. K's mental status exam, commenting that his responses to questions have ranged from "incoherent word salad" to "confused and disorganized." Although no behavioral issues or agitation are noted, he is reported to be irritable when redirected by staff members. The primary team has identified Mr. K as delirious, and their workup revealed a right lower lobe infiltrate on chest X-ray, leukocytosis, elevated creatinine, multiple electrolyte abnormalities, and lactatemia. You review his head CT, which demonstrates generalized parenchymal volume loss out of proportion to that expected at his age, but there is no acute pathology. Mr. K is being treated for an acute kidney injury, and is receiving antibiotics for a suspected aspiration pneumonia—although it is now resolved on a follow-up chest radiograph, and his leukocytosis is downtrending. His lab abnormalities have been corrected with intravenous fluids and supportive care. In the most recent medicine progress note, the problem list groups "delirium" and "schizoaffective disorder," with a plan to consult psychiatry given the patient's continued altered mental status and disorganization despite these medical improvements.

While reviewing the chart, you run through your differential diagnosis for AMS, and substance use and withdrawal is a critical consideration that can be overlooked in delirious patients. You find that Mr. K had a negative blood alcohol level and urine toxicology screen on arrival to the hospital. The team does not comment on alcohol use in the chart, and he is not being monitored for signs and symptoms of withdrawal, although you see he has been hypertensive and tachycardiac over his hospital course.

You decide to look for notes from prior hospital presentations to get a better sense of Mr. K's history, and see that he has had multiple emergency room visits for falls. On several of these visits, he was noted to have fallen while intoxicated, and presented with a highly elevated blood alcohol level. You return to Mr. K's labs and begin to look for any indirect biomarkers of chronic or heavy alcohol use that might be available—although nonspecific, these may provide clues when patients are unable to do so themselves. Mr. K has a macrocytosis on complete blood count, elevated liver enzymes, as well as hypoalbuminemia indicative of malnutrition and hepatic dysfunction. You check for thrombocytopenia, however his platelet count is normal. Continuing through the chart, you look for family contacts and cannot identify any, so you decide to seek collateral information from Mr. K's home care organization and outpatient psychiatrist. Mr. K's psychiatrist tells you that he has not seen the patient in months, but is unaware of any medical changes and believes that the patient has never had problems related to substance use. Mr. K's home aide is also uncertain about the amount of alcohol he uses, but does recall finding empty liquor bottles around his apartment.

You decide to gather more information from the primary team, and the resident reports that Mr. K has not demonstrated any signs of alcohol withdrawal. While the resident initially tells you that Mr. K does not have any history of substance use, he reluctantly acknowledges that the patient could not be interviewed at the time of admission, and the team did not obtain a substance use history. He is surprised to learn that Mr. K has presented to the hospital with falls and alcohol intoxication in the past. You consider the evidence from Mr. K's presentation—recent behavioral changes, altered mental status, aspiration, cerebral atrophy, and abnormal laboratory biomarkers—and grow increasingly concerned about unrecognized alcohol use and withdrawal. Although it may seem unlikely that heavy alcohol use would go undetected by a patient's physicians and caregiver, Mr. K is socially isolated, and alcohol use disorder is under-recognized and often unaddressed in the elderly [10]. You express your concern to the primary resident, and he says that Mr. K is "likely out of the withdrawal window" and does not feel it could be contributing to his clinical presentation. You use the opportunity to provide education on the protracted course of alcohol withdrawal in the elderly, explaining that it tends to present with more cognitive effects and AMS, sleepiness, and hypertension compared to what he may be accustomed to treating in younger adults [11].

You find Mr. K in his room, and he appears to have had a long period of neglect predating admission–he is unkempt, underweight, has poor dentition, and dirt under his nails. You wake him up, but he mumbles "go away" and immediately falls back asleep. You wake him again and orient him by introducing yourself, explaining your role as a psychiatric consultant, and that you wish to speak with him to better understand how you can help. Mr. K is able to remain alert and respond to questions only with near-continuous stimuli. He is disoriented to date, year, hospital, and city, is grossly inattentive and unable to participate in evaluation of other cognitive domains. You explain that he is in the hospital, and ask for his understanding of why he was admitted. Mr. K responds "I work at the hospital. I came here this morning to check in on things." Mr. K reports that he drinks "almost none… just two or three beers" every night, although you recognize that many patients underestimate or underreport their alcohol use. You ask if he ever drinks more than that, or if he also consumes other types of alcohol. He responds "I don't know, maybe vodka" and cannot provide further details. While attempting to gather more history, Mr. K's responses continue to be vague, filled with detail that is inconsistent with known reality and the external environment, and at times become incoherent.

Mr. K is not in frank alcohol withdrawal, but you remain concerned that he is particularly vulnerable to its cognitive effects given his poor health status and the possible effects of heavy chronic alcohol use on his brain. You think that he may have subtle withdrawal symptoms affecting his cognition, level of alertness and attention. Mr. K is more alert and engageable than had been described earlier in his hospital course, but he is remarkably confused, disoriented, has impaired memory and is confabulating. You consider "downstream" sequelae of heavy alcohol use, and you begin to suspect Wernicke encephalopathy—a neuropsychiatric consequence of thiamine deficiency related to chronic alcohol use or other causes of malnutrition. Wernicke encephalopathy is marked by ophthalmoplegia, ataxia, and altered mental status; however all three symptoms occur simultaneously in only a minority of cases, resulting in substantial underdiagnosis [12]. You glance through the chart looking for physical therapy assessments, and see Mr. K has not been out of bed since his admission. You and the nurse assist Mr. K in ambulating, and he is ataxic, with a tentative, broad-based gait. There is no characteristic horizontal nystagmus or ophthalmoplegia on exam, but your suspicion for Wernicke encephalopathy remains high given his history and presence of two symptoms.

You find the primary team and provide your assessment, recommending nutrition consultation, a brain MRI to correlate with your clinical diagnosis (evaluating for mammillary body and thalamic lesions), initiating a protocol to monitor and treat Mr. K for delayed or prolonged alcohol withdrawal, as well as administering high-dose parenteral thiamine (500 mg three times daily). You emphasize that Wernicke-Korsakoff syndrome is typically undertreated when identified, and explain that high-dose thiamine is critical for reversing the encephalopathy and reducing the risk for morbidity and developing Korsakoff's syndrome (also known as amnestic-confabulatory syndrome). You understand that identifying the key clinical signs and educating teams about the treatment of Wernicke-Korsakoff syndrome is an important role of the psychiatric consultant, and is significantly associated with patients receiving appropriate and necessary treatment [12, 13]. Expressing therapeutic optimism following this period of diagnostic and treatment confusion, you tell the primary team that thiamine may improve Mr. K's symptoms and minimize or prevent progression to irreversible cognitive impairment. You also emphasize that Mr. K's delirium is likely multifactorial in etiology, with contributions from the pneumonia and electrolyte abnormalities in addition to a thiamine deficiency, and that the neuropsychiatric effects of each of these conditions may persist beyond their treatment and apparent resolution. You encourage the team to continue to make efforts to identify next of kin, knowing that Mr. K may still have preexisting or progressive cognitive deficits despite treatment effects, and that he may need support in decision making around his care and safe disposition planning. You inform the team that psychiatry will follow Mr. K's progress closely, and will assist with managing alcohol withdrawal, behavioral symptoms, and engaging him with motivational interviewing and resources for substance use treatment as his mental status improves.

Appendix: Summary Table

	Problems	Strategies
• *Patient symptoms and behaviors*	• Acute changes in clinical presentation or protracted course of symptoms • Cognitive: Confusion, disorientation, impaired memory, inattention • Physical exam: Changes in level of consciousness, psychomotor agitation or retardation • Behavioral disturbances: Agitation, restlessness, combativeness, impulsivity	• Acute changes in level of consciousness, cognition, and behavior should always be treated as a medical emergency and evaluated appropriately • Consider withdrawal and intoxication, regardless of age and length of hospitalization • Ensure the patient's environment is safe and minimize hazards from rooms of confused, agitated, suicidal, and impulsive patients • Consider initiating medication for agitation or psychotic symptoms, target medication choice to treat the underlying etiology
• *Provider-patient dynamics*	• Psychiatric biases, inexperience, and frustration regarding a lack of diagnosis or improvement results in a separation of *psychiatric* and *medical* problems, resulting in subtle neglect of one or the other, misattribution of medical symptoms to psychiatric disorders, or overmedication • Lack of treatment options or patient disengagement contributes to parallel provider disengagement, hopelessness or avoidance of patient • Patient agitation and aggression leads to team feeling anxious, fearful, angry	• Provide diagnostic clarity and psychoeducation, explicitly identify symptoms that are or are not due to an underlying psychiatric disorder if known, guide management of psychotropic medications • Attempt to re-engage the team's curiosity and connectedness by clarifying or broadening the differential diagnosis when appropriate; provide concrete, actionable next steps for the team to take in the workup or in patient care • Acknowledge and empathize with provider fear and anxiety which can contribute to avoidance of the agitated patient; offer psychoeducation to reduce fear, biases or misperceptions related to patient behaviors; provide a stepped agitation management plan to address safety, team anxiety, and increase sense of control

	Problems	Strategies
• *Inter-provider and provider-family dynamics*	• Team has an unacknowledged hope that psychiatry will solve a complex diagnostic or treatment problem when feeling *stuck* or de-skilled with a challenging patient • Provider has underlying or unconscious wish for psychiatry to assume care of a demoralizing or anxiety-provoking case	• Set realistic expectations for what can be offered, while maintaining optimism that psychiatry can be helpful to the patient and team • Explicitly acknowledge when patients are challenging, partner with the team by following longitudinally and providing ongoing support, bolster the team's strengths while offering active interventions that can be made to assist with difficult patient behaviors and treatment engagement
• *Patient-provider barriers*	• Cognitive dysfunction, delirium, or reduced level of consciousness is interfering with patient-physician communication and patient's medical decision making	• Assist in identifying and addressing underlying etiologies of altered mental status • Remain available to assist in capacity evaluations around specific decisions, identify strategies to begin restoring capacity when possible • Identify and troubleshoot any factors preventing optimal communication (e.g., assistive devices for hearing and visual impairment, minimizing environmental distractions)
• *Hospital system barriers*	• Patient does not have available family, or is unable to identify individuals to serve as healthcare agents when incapacitated	• Assist in identifying next of kin, advise involvement of additional hospital services to navigate medico-legal or ethical challenges when appropriate (e.g., ethics consultation, hospital-based legal or administrative collaboration, patient advocacy services)

References

1. Bush G, Fink M, Petrides G, Dowling F, Francis A. Catatonia. I. Rating scale and standardized examination. Acta Psychiatr Scand. 1996;93:129–36.
2. Oldham MA, Lee HB. Catatonia Vis-à-Vis delirium: the significance of recognizing catatonia in altered mental status. Gen Hosp Psychiatry. 2015;37:554–9.
3. Grover S, Ghosh A, Ghormode D. Do patients of delirium have catatonic features? An exploratory study. Psychiatry Clin Neurosci. 2014;68:644–51.
4. Llesuy JR, Medina M, Jacobson K, Cooper JJ. Catatonia under-diagnosis in the general hospital. J Neuropsychiatry Clin Neurosci. 2018;30:145–51.
5. Llesuy JR, Coffey M, Jacobson KC, Cooper JJ. Suspected delirium predicts the thoroughness of catatonia evaluation. J Neuropsychiatry Clin Neurosci. 2017;29:148–54.
6. Perry PJ, Wilborn CA. Serotonin syndrome vs neuroleptic malignant syndrome: a contrast of causes, diagnoses, and management. Ann Clin Psychiatry. 2012;24:155–62.
7. Taylor MA, Fink M. Catatonia in psychiatric classification: a home of its own. Am J Psychiatry. 2003;160:1233–41.
8. Daniels J. Catatonia: clinical aspects and neurobiological correlates. J Neuropsychiatry Clin Neurosci. 2009;21:371–80.
9. Ananth J, Aduri K, Parameswaran S, Gunatilake S. Neuroleptic malignant syndrome: risk factors, pathophysiology, and treatment. Acta Neuropsychiatr. 2004;16:219–28.
10. Lehmann SW, Fingerhood M. Substance-use disorders in later life. N Engl J Med. 2018;379:2351–60.
11. Brower KJ, Mudd S, Blow FC, Young JP, Hill EM. Severity and treatment of alcohol withdrawal in elderly versus younger patients. Alcohol Clin Exp Res. 1994;18:196–201.
12. Isenberg-Grzeda E, Kutner HE, Nicolson SE. Wernicke-Korsakoff-syndrome: under-recognized and under-treated. Psychosomatics. 2012;53:507–16.
13. Nakamura ZM, Tatreau JR, Rosenstein DL, Park EM. Clinical characteristics and outcomes associated with high-dose intravenous thiamine administration in patients with encephalopathy. Psychosomatics. 2018;59:379–87.

Further Reading

Denysenko L, Sica N, Penders TM, Philbrick KL, Walker A, Shaffer S, Zimbrean P, Freudenreich O, Rex N, Carroll BT, Francis A. Catatonia in the medically ill: etiology, diagnosis, and treatment. The academy of consultation-liaison psychiatry evidence-based medicine subcommittee monograph. Ann Clin Psychiatry. 2018;30:140–55.

Substance Intoxication and Withdrawal

4

Kristopher A. Kast and Jonathan Avery

Your pager reads: "Suicidal and agitated polysubstance abuser."

This pager message succinctly condenses several questions for the consulting psychiatrist working with treatment teams caring for individuals with substance use and related disorders: Who are we treating? What are we treating? Are—and, if so, how are—these problematic behaviors related to substance use?

Substance use disorders (SUD) are common, complex, chronic, and relapsing neuropsychiatric disorders with well-described inherited risk, conserved neuropathology, and multiple effective treatment modalities [1, 2]. Individuals with substance use disorders are cared for by medical and surgical teams across every specialty and level of care. SUD-associated health consequences represent a substantial public health burden, including high emergency medical service utilization, infectious disease transmission, deleterious effects on every organ system, obstetrics and neonatal complications, and premature mortality [3, 4].

K. A. Kast (✉)
Department of Psychiatry and Behavioral Sciences,
Vanderbilt University Medical Center, Nashville, TN, USA
e-mail: kristopher.a.kast@vumc.org

J. Avery
Department of Psychiatry, NewYork-Presbyterian Hospital,
New York, NY, USA

A. Gorun et al. (eds.), *The Psychiatric Consult*,
https://doi.org/10.1007/978-3-031-26837-3_4

Importantly, stigma and unconscious bias against individuals with substance use disorders are prevalent among clinicians across specialties. As a group, physicians avoid working with the SUD population, are pessimistic about the efficacy of evidence-based treatment, and view individuals with SUD as poorly motivated, manipulative, of lower importance, and more dangerous or violent than other patients [5]. These attitudes lead to low provider empathy, reduced provider involvement, and depersonalized patient care [5].

The treatment team requesting consultation here uses a stigmatizing term to refer to the patient: "abuser." This term reflects historical diagnostic categories (separating physiological "dependence" from "abuse") meant to indicate severity of disordered behavior; these have since been removed in favor of less stigmatizing and more precise descriptive language [6, 7]. Wittingly or unwittingly, using the term "abuser" undermines the disease model of addiction, colloquially connoting volitional "bad" behavior driving recurrent substance use. This may affect the treatment team's ability to conceptualize the behavior as symptomatic of SUD and a target of treatment—rather than a moral failing outside the scope of medical practice. Further, the implicit view of the patient "behaving badly" in medical settings increases the risk of misdiagnosis, undertreatment, and subsequent medical complications—including post-discharge overdose.

The qualifier "polysubstance" is also prevalent in the general medical lexicon, serving as shorthand for multiple individual substance use disorders—implicitly and incorrectly suggesting that the specific diagnoses are less important data. Clarifying specific diagnoses for each substance category—identifying the current substance exposures and distinguishing use disorder from unhealthy use and episodic use—guides acute treatment and aftercare planning, and also offers an opportunity to engage the patient in a dialogue about their use, with the potential to motivate change. Further, using less-stigmatizing language in discussions with the team will also model respectful discourse that may re-humanize the patient in the treatment team's minds and refocus clinical attention on specific diagnoses requiring targeted treatment.

Clinical Scenario

You review the electronic medical record, finding that the patient—Ms. D—is a 28-year-old woman admitted to the general medical floor with a left upper-extremity skin and soft tissue infection requiring incision, drainage, and intravenous (IV) antibiotics. Ms. D is noted to have multiple puncture sites on her bilateral upper extremities of varying ages and stages of healing; she endorsed IV fentanyl use and unprescribed buprenorphine use to her medical team, but was not thought to be intoxicated or withdrawing on admission. Her routine urine toxicology screen showed only cannabinoids and she did not have a detectable blood alcohol level. Her physical examination and other routine screening labs were consistent with her presenting infection and had improved with treatment. HIV and viral hepatitis screening was negative. She has no prior records available, and the treatment team has not documented any other pertinent history.

The medical resident on the phone is clearly frustrated with the patient, expressing concern that Ms. D is manipulating their team by reporting pain that is out of proportion to the presenting problem (i.e., "she might be drug-seeking"). The resident also feels that the infectious site is improving and she may be ready for discharge from the medical floor soon—"so maybe we can transfer her to [inpatient] psych since she is suicidal?" The team has not clarified the patient's suicidal statements, noting that they heard about them from nursing staff. The nurses also report that she has been increasingly "agitated," though it is not immediately clear to you what is meant by the term.

"Agitation" is frequently a nonspecific catchall for difficult-to-control, treatment-interfering behaviors—especially when staff feel unsafe or directly threatened by the patient. Ensuring the safety of the staff, the milieu, and the patient is a primary goal of the consultation, and this is best accomplished by understanding the nature and etiology of the agitated behavior. Agitation has a broad diagnostic differential in the SUD population, with possible causes including intoxication and withdrawal states, undiagnosed or untreated medical comorbidity, undiagnosed or untreated psychiatric comorbidity, and problematic behaviors symptomatic of the SUD (e.g., attempting to leave the hospital against medical advice with a central venous catheter in place). Too often, implicit negative bias toward patients with SUD leads to the assumption that agitation reflects antisocial behavior.

Acknowledging and naming the felt distress of staff who are threatened by the "agitated" behavior may open the cognitive space for more detailed clarifying questions. Then identifying the specific behaviors of concern will allow you to be more helpful to both the team and the patient.

Scenario 1: Opioid Withdrawal

At the bedside, you find Ms. D sitting stooped over the edge of her bed with a bandaged arm guarding her abdomen. She is initially irritable and dismissive after you introduce yourself and your role: "I ask for pain medicine, and they think I'm crazy!"

You suspect that mutual frustration in the team (implicitly perceiving the patient as manipulative or deceptive) and the patient (experiencing pain that the team is reluctant to assess and treat) has led to an alliance rupture, impairing the dyad's ability to effectively communicate and pursue shared goals. You acknowledge and validate her frustration and experience of being unheard and dismissed, then add you hope to be helpful to her and her treatment team by clarifying and understanding her current experience—you ask for more information about her pain.

Her gaze is averted throughout much of the interview, but when she does make eye contact you notice lacrimation, frequent sniffling, and repeated wiping of her runny nose; she worries aloud about her frequent loose stools, noting that her team said "I don't have *C. diff.*" You ask her permission to assess her pupil size and find them to be quite dilated; her tremulous arms have prominent piloerection, as well.

You are concerned that the patient's pain and "drug-seeking" may reflect an unrecognized opioid withdrawal state. The resident's response to your questions before the consult suggested that they had not considered acute withdrawal, having been prematurely reassured by the available data: Ms. D's initial presentation in an asymptomatic state, a urine toxicology screen without opioids, and last reported use several days ago. However, routine urine immunohistochemical toxicology screens frequently do not assess for many synthetic opioids, and a withdrawal state is likely with her current symptoms [8, 9].

When you ask Ms. D about her prior experience with opioid withdrawal, she says, "what I'm feeling right now is a little like when I tried to come off oxycodone last year… but the last time I was *really* dope-sick was when I took Suboxone too soon after shooting fentanyl… I've been trying to detox' myself with the Suboxone, but I keep using again." Her pain is diffuse and musculoskeletal in nature, and has worsened with her sleep-onset insomnia—"I can't fall asleep, especially if I don't use… then I'm tired and in pain all day, I don't even want to go to work or meet up with friends anymore… I just stay in my apartment and think about how I haven't accomplished anything since college and how useless it feels to keep trying." Ms. D adds that she smokes cannabis some nights to help her fall asleep; she heard that it could also help her pain, but she is not sure it works for her.

Hearing her hopeless tone, you recall Ms. D's reported suicidal ideation. Expressed suicidal ideation may communicate a range of concerns from ambiguous distress (e.g., "If you discharge me, I'll kill myself") requiring clarification, to more specific symptomatology and suicidal risk associated with treatable psychiatric comorbidity (e.g., researching and/or planning for suicide by firearm in the context of a major depressive episode). Keeping in mind the high rate of comorbidity with other psychiatric disorders among SUD patients, you complete an assessment for additional features of a major depressive episode and rule out other potential etiologies, including adjustment disorder, bipolar depression, and post-traumatic stress disorder [10]. Aware that attempted and completed suicides are associated with intoxication states and SUD [11], you broaden your safety assessment and discover the patient's recent experience of an overdose where "I knew I could die if I did that much [fentanyl], but I didn't really care." She was resuscitated via intranasal naloxone administered by a friend who found her unresponsive at home. You consider this overdose a potential suicide attempt, since the desire to die (or suicidal intent) preceding opioid overdoses ranges on a continuum and is not a clear "yes-or-no" binary variable [12]. She has difficulty identifying social supports or other protections against suicide or overdose.

After completing your initial assessment, you share your impression with Ms. D by gathering her chaotic subjective experience into two diagnostic baskets: an opioid use disorder with current opioid withdrawal driving her pain, and a major depressive episode that may be opioid-induced or reflect an underlying primary major depressive disorder. You add that depressive symptoms are common when individuals enter treatment for opioid use disorder, and for some these resolve with initial stabilization—however, a significant group continues to experience depressive symptoms that warrant concurrent clinical attention and treatment with antidepressant therapy [11]. You also note that her infrequent cannabis use to manage her pain and insomnia does not appear to be impairing to her or meet the minimum of two criteria for a use disorder, though you worry about its effects on her mood and impulse control. Ms. D finds it helpful to connect her recurrent experience of diffuse pain and restless sleep to opioid withdrawal and agrees to initiate treatment for this.

The treatment team and nursing staff find it helpful to reframe the patient's problematic behaviors as expressions of distress in the setting of untreated opioid withdrawal, increasing empathic connection to her experience and reducing frustration. Ms. D is stabilized on combination buprenorphine-naloxone, with regular assessment of her symptoms by nursing staff using an objective scale. The initial alliance rupture begins to improve as Ms. D and her team move toward a common goal and her acute distress resolves.

You return the next day to reassess Ms. D and engage her in a discussion about her treatment goals using a motivational interviewing approach. You summarize and reflect her "change talk," highlighting her expressed internal motivation to reduce her fentanyl use. With Ms. D's permission, you share your recommendation to transition to maintenance pharmacotherapy for her opioid use disorder to reduce her risk of relapse and overdose.

You recommend transitioning to an inpatient psychiatric unit for further stabilization with antidepressant medication and psychotherapy in individual and group settings given the severity of her opioid use disorder, comorbid major depressive episode of unclear etiology, and significant safety concerns. You also discuss potential further SUD treatment in a residential, partial hospital, or intensive outpatient program to build skills for relapse prevention and initiate evidence-based psychosocial interventions that may be helpful to the patient in early recovery, such as motivational enhancement therapy, cognitive or dialectical behavior therapy, acceptance and commitment therapy, or 12-step peer support programs [13].

Since Ms. D has another day of antibiotic treatment, she asks for more time to consider these options before making a decision—but she thanks you, feeling helped by her work with you so far.

Scenario 2: Pregnant Patient with Substance Use Disorder

During your initial call with the treatment team, the resident also adds that Ms. D's newly discovered pregnancy "only makes matters worse—she kept asking if we were calling Child Protective Services and kicked us out of the room!"

The pregnant patient with SUD presents a complex ethical problem for clinicians. The overarching interests of the mother and the fetus are largely aligned, as engagement in prenatal care and treatment of the SUD lead to improved outcomes for both [14]. However, any substance use by the mother is potentially harmful to the fetus, and untreated SUD may impair a new mother's ability to provide a safe and adequate environment for growth and development after birth—thus, a mother's autonomy may come into conflict with the good of her child.

The role of Child Protective Services (CPS) is to assess the risk to a newborn child and optimize the home environment, whether that is determined to be with the mother, another family member, or in foster care. Clinicians are mandated reporters to CPS, and a positive toxicology screen in a new mother should trigger a CPS assessment—though the mandate varies significantly by state and clinicians must be familiar with relevant local legislation before making a referral [14]. This creates a complex motivational system for mothers with SUD. Added stigma and fear of losing custody of their child (and, in some states, additional criminal charges) may drive avoidance of prenatal care and hospital delivery, risking worsened outcomes for both the mother and her fetus. However, the possibility of receiving additional childcare supports and maintaining monitored custody that is contingent upon the mother's adherence to a treatment plan determined by CPS is a powerful motivation for engagement in SUD treatment and maintenance of recovery. The latter situation represents effective contingency management for the SUD while simultaneously realigning the interests of the maternal-fetal dyad.

Complicating the cognitive work involved in sorting through these ethical and motivational matrices, members of the treatment team may experience a range of emotions in response to Ms. D's pregnancy and the prospect of a CPS report—including anger, guilt, fear, anxiety, and conflicted tension of varying intensity. Acknowledging, naming, and validating the mixed and often conflicting emotional responses may helpfully contain any sense of overwhelm. This allows cognitive space for organizing conflicting ethical and legal considerations and allowing for clear communication and treatment planning. Further, attending to both the emotional and cognitive conflicts may be extraordinarily helpful to the strained alliance between Ms. D and the treatment team—and ensure everyone involved is attending to the interests of both the mother and her fetus.

On bedside assessment, you (again) find Ms. D sitting on the edge of her bed with stooped posture and a bandaged arm guarding her abdomen. She is apprehensive when you introduce yourself and your role, demanding to know if you are "here to see if I'm fit to be a mother?" You acknowledge and validate her concern and clearly state the limits of confidentiality specific to your local jurisdiction's mandated reporting, which typically is not in effect antenatally. You also ask open-ended questions about the patient's pain.

As in the first scenario, you diagnose acute opioid withdrawal evidenced by her dilated pupils, piloerection, lacrimation, rhinorrhea, diarrhea, restlessness, and diffuse musculoskeletal pain. In sharing this diagnosis with the patient, you ask permission to share additional information about opioid withdrawal in pregnancy. You review the risks of fetal distress, premature labor, and spontaneous abortion [14], and recommend stabilization using an opioid agonist (methadone or buprenorphine) with subsequent maintenance pharmacotherapy. Considering this information, Ms. D asks, "But isn't exposing the baby to another opioid risky, too? I want whatever is safest."

After reflecting back her clear motivation to protect her fetus, you reframe her question as balancing the risk of a stable controlled dose of a prescribed opioid against the risk of untreated withdrawal and fetal distress. You query her understanding of this risk calculus, and further highlight the subsequent risk of untreated opioid use disorder, including relapse with repeated fluctuating states of intoxication and withdrawal, as well as exposure to teratogenic adulterant substances mixed with illicit opioids. And finally, you review the known benefits of opioid agonist pharmacotherapy in pregnancy, including improved maternal health and nutrition, reduced obstetric complications, improved health of the newborn at delivery, and enhanced ability to parent and provide an adequate home environment postpartum [13, 14].

Hearing your recommendations, Ms. D asks to discuss her treatment with the consulting obstetrics team to ensure she has the thoughts of all involved physicians. You touch base with the primary treatment team and the obstetrics team, reviewing the diagnosis and treatment recommendations; these are agreed upon and reinforced to the patient by each team.

Ms. D agrees to stabilization with the "mono" buprenorphine product, without the addition of a naloxone deterrent, given theoretical concerns for teratogenicity [14]. She is encouraged by the possibility of improved perinatal pain control, shorter postpartum hospital length of stay, and less severe neonatal opioid withdrawal syndrome compared with methadone [13, 14]. She also finds office-based treatment preferable to the intensive engagement with a methadone treatment program.

With stabilization, Ms. D's mild subsyndromal depressive symptoms improve, and she clarifies her previous vague suicidal statements as "not knowing how else to express that I was feeling trapped and without help." She cites her relationship to her fetus and anticipation of being a mother as protective against suicide.

She also asks appropriate questions around her occasional cannabis use, noting that she had heard of its antiemetic effects for *hyperemesis gravidarum*—"and I've heard it's pretty safe in pregnancy." You provide information on the exposure of the fetus to both carbon monoxide and delta-9-tetrahydrocannabinol (THC) when pregnant women smoke cannabis products, since both easily cross the placenta, and the documented risks of stillbirth and neurodevelopmental deficits found in children prenatally exposed [14]. You add that cannabidiol (CBD) products may also confer risk to the developing fetus [15] and that even though CBD is not assessed on most toxicology screens, CBD products do contain detectable levels of THC, posing a legal risk to the patient should she be screened at the time of delivery [16].

Over the remaining days of her hospitalization, Ms. D educates herself on the local mandated reporting laws and role of CPS. She feels motivated to engage actively in her SUD treatment to protect her fetus and her ability to maintain custody, planning to also participate in group therapy and a peer-support group for mothers with SUD through the hospital's outpatient department.

Scenario 3: Alcohol-Induced Psychotic Disorder

During your initial call with the treatment team, the resident is adamant that Ms. D should be transferred to inpatient psychiatry, "since she probably has schizophrenia—she's hearing voices and is extremely paranoid—and she's never taken an antipsychotic or seen a psychiatrist before!"

This additional information about acute, new-onset psychotic symptoms shifts your differential diagnosis. On bedside assessment, your initial suspicion for delirium is not supported by the patient's intact arousal and attention—as well as her flawless execution of the clock-draw task, after some encouragement to participate. You do notice some tremulousness as she handles the pen and paper, as well as diaphoretic skin with mild tachycardia and hypertension displayed on her monitor.

Suspecting concurrent alcohol withdrawal, you ask the patient about her use—but her significant paranoia and hallucinatory experiences limit her reporting ("I'm not sure I can trust you… the voice is telling me you're in on it, too!"). Re-reviewing her routine laboratories (which included a negative blood alcohol level on arrival), you notice that she has an elevated mean corpuscular volume (MCV) and aspartate aminotransferase (AST), both suggestive markers of heavy alcohol use [9].

You share your diagnostic impression with the treatment team—an alcohol-induced psychotic disorder (formerly "alcoholic hallucinosis") in the setting of alcohol withdrawal—and clarify the distinction between this diagnosis and *delirium tremens*, given the lack of concurrent delirium or severe dysautonomia. In addition to urgent neuroimaging to rule-out an acute neuroaxial process driving her psychosis, you also advise the team to treat the patient empirically with lorazepam while assessing her response using a validated objective alcohol withdrawal scale and trending vital signs. You reinforce that benzodiazepine treatment will reduce the risk of withdrawal seizures in the first 24 h and prevent progression to delirium, which typically develops at 72–96 h [17]. You also discuss the potential utility of obtaining additional biomarkers of heavy alcohol use, including gamma-glutamyltransferase (GGT), which may be more sensitive than MCV or AST in detecting alcohol use disorder; urinary ethyl glucuronide or ethyl sulfate, extremely sensitive markers of alcohol exposure in the prior 2–3 days; carbohydrate-deficient transferrin, a marker of heavy alcohol use within the past 2 weeks; or phosphatidylethanol, a marker of heavy use over the prior 2–3 weeks.

On reassessment the next day, Ms. D is calm and cooperative with stabilized vital signs and remitted psychosis. She is better able to engage in a full assessment, including recanting her previously reported suicidality and clarifying her substance use history, revealing difficulty with cutting back on her daily alcohol and episodic opioid use. She agrees to convert the total dose of lorazepam required to stabilize her alcohol withdrawal in the first 24 h to a short taper over the next several days. You also engage her in a discussion of available pharmacotherapy for alcohol use disorder and her comorbid opioid use disorder, recommending long-acting injectable naltrexone given its dual indication for both, alongside intensive psychosocial treatment.

Ms. D also reports concern about her increasing cannabis use, using an electronic cigarette or "vaping" device, since she has sometimes experienced similar paranoid thoughts and auditory hallucinations on her heaviest-use days. She has also been concerned about the reports of deaths due to vaping-induced lung injury, which she knows has been most closely linked to THC-containing products [18]—but she has had difficulty cutting back or stopping her use despite these concerns. Reinforcing her engagement and active motivation for change, you share information about cannabis use disorder and the connection between higher THC-content and psychotic symptoms during intoxication [19]. You also provide a reflective statement to Ms. D, noting that she has experienced psychotic symptoms both in the hospital during alcohol withdrawal and when using cannabis heavily; then you pause, inviting her response. Appearing tentative, Ms. D worries aloud if "I might be schizophrenic… [the treatment team] asked me if I'd ever been diagnosed."

Clarifying that she has never experienced psychotic symptoms outside an intoxication or withdrawal state, you educate her about her diagnosis—substance-induced psychotic disorder—and its relationship to schizophrenia-spectrum disorders. You share that chronic cannabis use is considered a risk factor for developing a primary schizophrenia-spectrum disorder, a twofold increased risk compared with nonusing individuals, and add that current recommendations are to abstain from use to reduce this risk [20]. Since Ms. D reports symptoms of a cannabis use disorder, you recommend targeted treatment alongside her comorbid alcohol and opioid use disorders. You highlight that although there are no FDA-approved medications for cannabis use disorder, psychosocial treatments are effective and some medications have limited evidence for helping with cannabis withdrawal symptoms and even reducing use [21]. You also recommend engaging in psychiatric treatment for monitoring of her now remitted psychotic symptoms, and reinforce the availability of effective treatments should psychosis recur. This final recommendation is motivated by the high risk of transition to a schizophrenia-spectrum disorder in individuals with substance-induced psychosis, with 10–20% conversion for alcohol and up to 46% for cannabis-induced symptoms [19].

Ms. D thanks you for your help, using language that suggests significant motivation to change her patterns of use and engage in treatment after completing her medical hospitalization.

Appendix: Summary Table

	Problems	Strategies
• Patient symptoms and behaviors	• Misidentified intoxication or withdrawal states • Underlying medical or psychiatric comorbidity • In-hospital substance use	• Assist with diagnostic clarification using objective measures of withdrawal (e.g., Clinical Opiate Withdrawal Scale, COWS; Objective Alcohol Withdrawal Scale, OAWS) and/or distinguishing signs and symptoms of intoxication from withdrawal • Assist in selecting appropriate toxicology assessment (e.g., expanding to synthetic opioids, specific benzodiazepines, GC/MS confirmatory testing) and interpreting results • Provide guidance in evidence-based treatment for intoxication and withdrawal states specific to the underlying substances • Assist in assessment of reported medical or psychiatric symptoms, broadening differential diagnoses • Assist team in ensuring patient safety, removing access to further substances, and repairing therapeutic alliance between patient and team
• Provider-patient dynamics	• Provider and patient experience misaligned goals, struggling for control over care, and treatment planning • Patient and provider slip into implicit roles of the untrustworthy reporter and the suspicious detective, respectively	• Provide motivational interviewing interventions, modeling evocation of ambivalence, shared decision-making, and approaches to conflicts between patient autonomy and physicianly beneficence • Directly address the implicit assumptions around misreporting and model an alternative approach with healthy trust of the patient's experience balanced by respectful curiosity around conflicting data

	Problems	Strategies
• Inter-provider and provider-family dynamics	• Treatment team experiences decreased ownership of the SUD patient's symptoms and treatment, disengaging from diagnostic assessment, treatment planning, and/or requesting transfer to other providers • Treatment team over-identifies with well-meaning significant others, all together responding to the "righting reflex" to correct or control the patient's behavior	• Assist in broadening differential diagnoses to include problems within the team's expertise, and provide support in treatment planning for those aspects of treatment where the team feels de-skilled • Assist in assessing appropriate level-of-care for the patient's entire clinical presentation, providing reasoning to support the patient's continued medical admission or appropriate transfer to other settings (e.g., inpatient psychiatry, detoxification unit, or residential SUD treatment) • Consider continuing to follow and consult on the patient after evaluation to collaborate and provide team with support throughout the admission • Assist the team and significant others in managing the righting reflex, providing education around more effective approaches to ambivalence while acknowledging the place of caring concern underlying their attempts at control

	Problems	Strategies
• Patient-provider barriers	• Implicit bias against individuals with SUD leads to low provider engagement • Stigmatizing language is unwittingly used by the team, leading to conflict or patient disengagement • Prior negative experiences in healthcare environments leads patient to have low trust and poor initial alliance with the treatment team	• Recognize low provider engagement and assist in re-engaging teams in the patient's care, providing helpful reframing of the presenting problems and available effective treatments • Formal educational interventions on implicit bias among clinicians can be effective in improving attitudes; however, this may be less effective in the context of a specific consultation • Model use of less stigmatizing language ("person with opioid use disorder" instead of "opiate addict") in interactions with patients and teams • Recognize a poor therapeutic alliance and intervene; ask about and validate prior negative experiences; ask the patient what changes might allow the possibility of an improved experience here and now

	Problems	Strategies
• Hospital system barriers	• Low availability of treatment resources after discharge • Vulnerability to treatment drop-out in transitions from the hospital to the next level of care • Felt pressure to decrease length-of-stay, risking discharge prior to stabilization • Hospital rules/policies limiting patient autonomy (e.g., prohibiting smoke breaks, absences from the floor, required hospital gowns)	• Acknowledge treatment scarcity and provide support to teams in identifying appropriate discharge planning for ongoing management of the SUD • Offer resources directly to the patient, including online databases of peer support groups, hotlines, and low-barrier care (e.g, walk-in clinics) • Assist in risk assessment around discharge planning and recommended length of inpatient treatment for SUD-specific states (withdrawal, titration of pharmacotherapy, etc.) • Provide harm-reduction measures to the patient, including naloxone rescue kits with training in appropriate use and resources for safe injection practices (e.g., needle exchange or safe-injection programs) • Assist teams and staff in navigating complex risk calculus around restrictive hospital rules/policies, ensuring inclusion of the risk of patient elopement and/or unplanned discharge prior to completing treatment for their presenting medical problem • Consider creative solutions to manage patient discomfort while respecting hospital policies and the values underlying them (e.g., ensuring patient and staff safety)

References

1. Volkow ND, Boyle M. Neuroscience of addiction: relevance to prevention and treatment. Am J Psychiatry. 2018;175(8):729–40.
2. Koob GF. Neurobiology of addiction. In: Galanter M, Kleber HD, Brady KT, editors. Textbook of substance abuse treatment. 5th ed. Washington, DC: American Psychiatric Publishing; 2015.
3. Crum RM. The epidemiology of substance use disorders. In: Miller SC, Fiellin DA, Rosenthal R, Saitz R, editors. The ASAM principles of addiction medicine, vol. 6. Philadelphia: Wolters Kluwer; 2019.
4. Kunz K. The addiction medicine physician as a change agent for prevention and public health. In: Miller SC, Fiellin DA, Rosenthal R, Saitz R, editors. The ASAM principles of addiction medicine, vol. 6. Philadelphia: Wolters Kluwer; 2019.
5. Avery JD, Avery JJ. The stigma of addiction: an essential guide. Cham: Springer; 2019.
6. Saitz R, Miller SC, Fiellin DA. Recommended use of terminology in addiction medicine. In: Miller SC, Fiellin DA, Rosenthal R, Saitz R, editors. The ASAM principles of addiction medicine, vol. 6. Philadelphia: Wolters Kluwer; 2019.
7. American Psychiatric Publishing. Substance-related and addictive disorders. In: Diagnostic and statistical manual of mental disorders, vol. 5. Arlington: American Psychiatric Publishing; 2013.
8. Shorter D, Kosten TR. The pharmacology of opioids. In: Galanter M, Kleber HD, Brady KT, editors. Textbook of substance abuse treatment. 5th ed. Washington, DC: American Psychiatric Publishing; 2015.
9. Merlin JS, Warner EA, Starrels JL. Laboratory assessment. In: Miller SC, Fiellin DA, Rosenthal R, Saitz R, editors. The ASAM principles of addiction medicine, vol. 6. Philadelphia: Wolters Kluwer; 2019.
10. Avery JD, Barnhill JW. Co-occurring mental illness and substance use disorders: a guide to diagnosis and treatment. Arlington: American Psychiatric Association; 2018.
11. Nunes EV, Weiss RD. Co-occurring mood and substance use disorders. In: Miller SC, Fiellin DA, Rosenthal R, Saitz R, editors. The ASAM principles of addiction medicine, vol. 6. Philadelphia: Wolters Kluwer; 2019.
12. Connery HS, Taghian N, Kim J. Suicidal motivations reported by opioid overdose survivors: a cross-sectional study of adults with opioid use disorder. Drug Alcohol Depend. 2019;5:205.
13. Renner JA, Levounis P, LaRose AT. Office-based buprenorphine treatment of opioid use disorder, vol. 2. Arlington: American Psychiatric Publishing; 2019.
14. Weaver MF, Jones HE, Wunsch MJ. Alcohol and other drug use in pregnancy: management of the mother and child. In: Miller SC, Fiellin DA, Rosenthal R, Saitz R, editors. The ASAM principles of addiction medicine, vol. 6. Philadelphia: Wolters Kluwer; 2019.

15. Fish EW, Murdaugh LB, Zhang C. Cannabinoids exacerbate alcohol teratogenesis by a CB1-Hedgehog interaction. Sci Rep. 2019;9(1):16057.
16. Spindle TR, Cone EJ, Kuntz D, et al. Urinary pharmacokinetic profile of cannabinoids following administration of vaporized and oral cannabidiol and vaporized CBD-dominant cannabis. J Anal Toxicol. 2020;44(2):109–25.
17. Wartenberg AA. Management of alcohol intoxication and withdrawal. In: Miller SC, Fiellin DA, Rosenthal R, Saitz R, editors. The ASAM principles of addiction medicine, vol. 6. Philadelphia: Wolters Kluwer; 2019.
18. Centers for Disease Control and Prevention (CDC). Outbreak of lung injury associated with the use of e-cigarette, or vaping, products. Online publication. https://www.cdc.gov/tobacco/basic_information/e-cigarettes/severe-lung-disease.html. Accessed 21 Nov 2019.
19. Ziedonis D, Fan X, Larkin C. Co-occuring addiction and psychotic disorders. In: Miller SC, Fiellin DA, Rosenthal R, Saitz R, editors. The ASAM principles of addiction medicine, vol. 6. Philadelphia: Wolters Kluwer; 2019.
20. Fischer B, Russell C, Sabioni P. Lower-risk cannabis use guidelines: a comprehensive update of evidence and recommendations. Am J Public Health. 2017;107(8):e1–e12.
21. Kelly MA, Levin FR. Treatment of cannabis use disorder. In: Galanter M, Kleber HD, Brady KT, editors. Textbook of substance abuse treatment. 5th ed. Washington, DC: American Psychiatric Publishing; 2015.

Human Immunodeficiency Virus (HIV)

5

Jessica Spellun and Chloe Nims

Your pager reads: "The patient isn't eating".

This request for a psychiatric consult arrives, like many, not in the form of a question but of a chief complaint. A nonspecific behavior is described, containing both an implied suggestion of an underlying psychiatric cause as well as a request for help in management. To perform a consultation that is useful for the team, you will not just need to determine whether there is a psychiatric diagnosis contributing to this presentation and if there are modifiable behavioral factors, you will also need to understand how the interdisciplinary team understands the patient's behavior and how it may be impacting their interactions with the patient. If the patient's behavior is viewed as self-defeating, does the consult request reflect provider discomfort with feeling thwarted? Are there broader concerns related to adherence? Is the behavior a barrier to discharge planning? Your goal will be to establish the acute needs of the interdisciplinary team and the patient as well as to help identify contributions that relate to patient-team-hospital dynamics or hospital systems-based issues.

J. Spellun (✉) · C. Nims
Department of Psychiatry, NewYork-Presbyterian Hospital/
Weill Cornell Medicine, New York, NY, USA
e-mail: jes9244@med.cornell.edu

A. Gorun et al. (eds.), *The Psychiatric Consult*,
https://doi.org/10.1007/978-3-031-26837-3_5

Clinical Scenario

You review the chart of the patient, Mr. R, looking for clues to the underlying etiology, possible risks or medical sequelae stemming from his decline in appetite before calling the team back. You find that Mr. R is HIV positive and has been admitted for recurrent respiratory infections, unexplained weight loss, and fatigue. When you speak to the medical resident by phone, you learn that there have been daily reports from nursing staff that Mr. R is requiring a lot of their time and encouragement because he is refusing to eat. You sense frustration in the resident's voice as he reports that Mr. R's hospital course has been prolonged because of his refusal to take in adequate nutrition. As you attempt to clarify details of his behavior and mental status exam findings, the resident interrupts and bluntly states that they have excluded or treated any possible medical cause of Mr. R's failure to thrive, and that their team feels he may have a psychiatric illness that needs treatment. The resident tells you he needs to take an urgent call and, before hanging up the phone, apologizes for asking you to see such a "difficult patient."

Scenario 1: HIV and Major Depressive Disorder

In your initial review of Mr. R's chart, you learn that he was sent to the emergency room by a community primary care physician 7 days ago due to concern about an unintentional 40-pound weight loss and fatigue over a 3-month period. He is in his mid-40s, is married, and was previously employed in construction. His unexplained weight loss occurred in the context of a newly diagnosed HIV infection and sporadic medical follow-up. Initial blood work results are consistent with new untreated HIV infection and show a CD4 count of 350 cells/mm^3 and a viral load of 22,000 copies/mL in addition to a mild leukopenia and anemia. You see that the primary team has done a thorough medical workup including additional laboratory and imaging studies to rule out medical causes for weight loss—including, but not limited to, malignancy, infection, and toxic and metabolic disturbances. His respiratory infection has resolved with antibiotics. You check the medication administration history and see that there are intermittent entries stating that Mr. R "refused medications." As you conceptualize the case, you consider utilizing a screening tool such as the Hospital Anxiety and Depression Scale (HADS) to help identify the presence of anxiety and depression in the setting of symptom overlap with comorbid medical conditions, such as HIV [1].

You decide you would like to understand in more detail how Mr. R has been engaging with other team members. You attempt to call the resident again, but he is unavailable. You head to the unit to speak with nursing staff. You learn that Mr. R's nurses have become increasingly frustrated by his seeming total disinterest in eating. They are beginning to lose patience with the amount of time it takes to encourage him to eat and to take medications. They note that his wife has frequently brought in his favorite meals from home, and that Mr. R tends to become more withdrawn when she is visiting and declines her food. You notice that they seem to align and identify with his wife, frequently commenting on the fact that she is "a saint" for caring for him when he can be "so difficult." Nursing staff also comment on how pointless it has become to struggle with him over eating and that they believe he would fare better in a psychiatric unit. They quote him as saying that there is "no point" in eating and that he "doesn't deserve" the care they are providing, and they wonder whether he is at risk of acting on his feelings by harming himself. They seem worried. You take note of their conflicting statements regarding concern for his safety and a seeming desire to shift the burden of care to another service.

When you arrive to Mr. R's room, he is lying in bed, staring ahead with a female visitor seated next to him. She introduces herself as Mrs. R, his wife, and rolls her eyes wishing you luck before excusing herself from the room. Mr. R stoically avoids eye contact with you during introductions before eventually settling in to answer your questions. He endorses a history of recurrent major depressive episodes throughout his adult life, with one prior suicide attempt that required psychiatric hospitalization. He describes feeling more depressed since he was laid off from work 6 months ago. He has lost interest in food and has felt more and more fatigued. Mr. R relays that in an attempt to self-soothe he began to visit prostitutes. He tells you he is ashamed to admit that he did not use condoms, which led to his HIV infection. Upon testing positive 3 months ago he disclosed his status to his wife, whose initial shock and denial was followed by anger, sense of betrayal, and fear for her own health. This only compounded the marital conflict that had begun with the stress of his unemployment. He quietly berates himself, lamenting how "stupid" he has been for ruining everything that was good in his life, and he breaks down sobbing. Mr. R tells you that he does not know if he can live with himself if his wife has contracted HIV.

You note some negative judgment toward Mr. R in your countertransference, which is in tension with your feelings of empathy evoked by his deep shame and guilt. You recognize how these feelings may also be reflected in the nurses' alignment with Mrs. R's anger and impatience as they also try to protect him. You wonder whether the countertransference experienced by providers mirrors Mr. R's internal experience of self-directed anger and hopelessness. You find yourself pulled to comfort him and alleviate feelings of isolation in his self-reproach. You share what you have learned about sex-seeking behaviors in depression as a means to temporarily increase self-esteem—deflated for Mr. R after losing his employment—and how cognitive **distortions** and negative self-appraisals associated with depression correlate with decreased use of safer sex measures [2].

Your assessment interview combined with Mr. R's scores on the HADS screening tool reveals that he is experiencing a major depressive episode as defined by DSM5 criteria [3] and that this has reduced his motivation for adherence to prescribed antiretroviral therapy (ART). The societal stigma and marginalization of persons experiencing HIV aligns with his internal self-reprimanding and has furthered his isolation from social supports, his wife, and his primary care physician [4]. He reports near-constant thoughts that everyone would be better off if he were dead and describes fantasizing about ending his life. Your evaluation includes an assessment of Mr. R's safety: he reveals that his suicidal fantasies have included purchasing a firearm, hanging himself, and drinking alcohol and cutting his wrists in a hotel, where no one will intervene.

Given the well-established higher rates of depression in HIV-positive populations [4], and the association between depression and reduced adherence to ART [5], you emphasize with Mr. R the need to reengage with psychiatric care. You attempt to instill hope about the psychotherapeutic interventions available for acceptance and adjustment to his HIV status, in addition to evidence-based psychotherapy options for depression. You notice a shift in Mr. R's affect as you speak and you encourage him to express his fears about acknowledging and learning how to manage life with a potentially life-threatening chronic illness. Your empathic responses will help Mr. R to verbalize, express, and tolerate his emotions so he can then begin to learn to develop self-empathy through mirroring [6].

An appreciation of the safety risks and the success of treatment interventions thus far should help to guide you in determining next steps. Mr. R is at an acutely elevated risk of harming himself and is having difficulties engaging with outpatient medical and psychiatric care. Considering these factors, you recommend inpatient psychiatric hospitalization to the patient and primary medical team. As there is sometimes a delay in obtaining an inpatient psychiatric bed in your institution, you recommend that Mr. R begin treatment with a Selective Serotonin Reuptake Inhibitor (SSRI) and you recommend escitalopram or sertraline, which have fewer drug–drug interactions with the common ART medications. You also consider bupropion because of the theoretical benefit to HIV-positive patients, given the known reduction in dopaminergic activity in mood-critical brain areas resulting from HIV infection [7]. In your medication decision-making, you consider that Mr. R has previously experienced remission from major depressive episodes with SSRIs, and that several commonly used ART medications affect bupropion metabolism. You also consider Mr. R's low weight and appetite changes and have some concerns that this may be worsened by the stimulant-like effects of bupropion, which also carries an increased risk for seizures when used in underweight individuals [8]. You provide the team with education as to the benefits of modafinil or stimulants in treating comorbid depression, fatigue, and HIV [9]. You also inform them of the risks of appetite suppression and seizures when considering use of stimulants in this population [9].

Scenario 2: HIV and Severe and Persistent Mental Illness

You complete a review of Mr. R's chart and note that he is a 62-year-old man with a history of schizophrenia, former IV heroin use currently on methadone maintenance, and chronic street homelessness. He has extensive chart notes in your system. Psychiatric emergency room notes indicate that his longest period of adherence to neuroleptics and ART was during the time he spent in prison after violating probation related to multiple nonviolent misdemeanor charges. In addition to HIV/Acquired Immune Deficiency Syndrome (AIDS), he has comorbid type 2 diabetes mellitus, hyperlipidemia, hypertension, and coronary artery disease. He is noted to have only sporadic follow-up with outpatient medical and psychiatric care.

Mr. R was brought in to the emergency room after he was found muttering incoherently to himself on a street corner in the middle of winter, with scant and tattered clothing. Initial workup revealed a CD4 count of 42 cells/mm^3 and a high viral load in addition to evidence of chronic undernutrition, acid–base imbalance and subsequent detection of Pneumocystis (PCP) pneumonia on chest imaging. He has had a long hospitalization and notes suggest initial altered mental status and somnolence and you suspect he may have been delirious at time of presentation. You speak with the medical resident who explains that they have not found a clear medical cause for Mr. R's diminished interest in food and seeming fatigue, which is out of proportion for that which is expected during recovery from pneumonia. He emphasizes that this is a patient with schizophrenia who has appeared internally preoccupied throughout his long admission to their service, and suggests that Mr. R may need to be psychiatrically hospitalized. The resident adds that the team restarted Mr. R on haloperidol, which was ordered during his last admission but which he routinely declines when the nurses bring him the pill. You clarify with the team that one of their consult requests is for the transfer of Mr. R to inpatient psychiatry.

The physical therapy (PT) and occupational therapy (OT) teams are recommending disposition to a subacute rehab, as Mr. R has become physically deconditioned. It is also noted that he may require longer-term placement in a skilled nursing facility, given concerns about his ability to care for his basic medical and daily living needs. Occupational therapy notes after medical treatment and apparent resolution of delirium reveal a Montreal Cognitive Assessment (MoCA) of 18/30 along with deficits in activities of daily living, memory, multistep commands, and executive function. Neurology has been consulted during the admission and imaging was done, which shows mild generalized parenchymal volume loss and no evidence of intracranial central nervous system infection, malignancy, or other space occupying lesions. The neurology team noted that there were a number of factors contributing to his poor cognitive performance including the untreated schizophrenia, the sequelae of delirium, and HIV-Associated Neurocognitive Disorder (HAND)—specifically HIV dementia from nonadherence to ART. Mr. R has been started on an antiretroviral agent that has good CNS penetrance and low risk for neurotoxicity with the hope of restoring some neurocognitive functioning over time.

You meet with Mr. R and find him to be alert, oriented to person and place, and pleasant and attentive, and you note that he has mild perioral movements indicative of tardive dyskinesia. Mr. R provides disorganized, tangential answers to questions consistent with a formal thought disorder. Nonetheless he can meaningfully convey the outlines of his long-standing experience of homelessness and convey his wish to avoid psychiatric care and the particularly bothersome side effects of antipsychotic medications. You note his ambivalence while making efforts to engage him around collaborative goal setting. You ask his permission to discuss alternative neuroleptics with more favorable side effect profiles. Given the increased risk of extrapyramidal symptoms (EPS) in patients with HIV [10] you are considering the second-generation antipsychotics with less dopamine blockade activity. Mr. R ultimately agrees to a change when you align with his treatment goals and his desire to avoid rehospitalization. You hope to identify important community contacts who might be able to support adherence to treatment in the hospital and acceptance of the ultimate disposition plan. Mr. R relays that he lost contact with his family many decades ago and that his main social supports are the counselor at his methadone program and the pastor at the church soup kitchen he frequents.

Mr. R can provide you with limited but accurate information about his illness, hospital course, and conversations about discharge planning. He expresses appreciation for his medical team and for the social workers who are helping to arrange aftercare. He acknowledges that he is feeling physically unwell and unable to protect himself from danger on the streets anymore. You complete a full psychiatric evaluation and he does not endorse mood symptoms or suicidality. Intermittently throughout the interview, he appears to respond to internal stimuli and mutters to himself. He does not show impairments in attention on mini mental status exam. His lunch tray arrives during the interview and you find that he attempts to eat, but struggles with fine motor movements and praxis while using his utensils before losing interest and dismissing the hospital food as being "gross." In noting the fine motor deficits in combination with the cognitive features of apathy and lethargy, you begin to conceptualize Mr. R's failure to thrive as multifactorial, reflecting the overlap of HIV dementia, schizophrenia, and side effects of antipsychotic medication.

The most recent social work notes document that most of the subacute rehab facilities in your area, which accept Mr. R's managed medicaid plan, have rejected his application. You wonder whether your thoughts that this is related to stigma around his severe and persistent mental illness (SPMI) , substance use, criminal justice involvement, and AIDS are justified or overly cynical. You think about the hardships Mr. R must have endured in his life compounded by the limited understanding he must often face in institutional settings of the morbidity that accrues in patients with SPMI and HIV. You consider the impact of executive functioning impairments, disorganization, and the cycles of mistrust and discrimination due to chronic psychosis that can lead to patient, provider, and societal behaviors that impede treatment and access to public services and medical care [11, 12]. You remind yourself of the known higher rates of HIV in people experiencing SPMI and substance use disorders, and also of the challenges to adherence for treatable illness imposed by poverty, lack of housing, associated trauma, and all that it takes to survive [11, 12]. You begin to appreciate how easily the challenges faced by the patient could overwhelm providers, and in an attempt to defend against this experience, how providers might be led to conceptualize the patient's behaviors as volitional.

You return to the team and actively empathize with and validate their frustrations in establishing a discharge plan for Mr. R, highlighting his complex needs and the excellent care that they have provided him during his hospitalization. You provide psychoeducation around the patient's psychotic symptoms and emphasize that they do not pose a degree of risk that would warrant psychiatric hospitalization. You add that his difficulties in caring for his basic needs are multifactorial and that antipsychotic medications are less effective in targeting negative symptoms than positive, the former being more likely to contribute to poor self-care. You emphasize the use of patient-centered language and the fact that Mr. R does demonstrate a basic understanding of his current medical needs. You underscore the importance of establishing and following his wishes pertaining to quality of life, treatment options, and setting.

You provide the team with recommendations, including the suggestion that interdisciplinary collaboration occur to determine the best disposition plan to allow Mr. R to live the remainder of his life according to his wishes. You suggest that this may include involving chaplain services and contacting the pastor at his soup kitchen. You also recommend that a palliative care consult be considered in an effort to expand support for his emotional and spiritual well-being as well as his comfort and medical needs. You emphasize that the psychiatry team will continue to follow and assist with this psychiatrically and medically complicated patient. A week later, you learn that Mr. R's pastor is now visiting him in the hospital and has been instrumental in helping to facilitate a transfer to a long-term nursing facility where he plans to continue to visit Mr. R and bring favored meals from the soup kitchen menu.

Scenario 3: HIV and Post-Traumatic Stress Disorder

During your initial chart review, you notice that multiple notes reference that this 25-year-old patient identifies as a transgender woman (with male sex assigned at birth). Your electronic medical record is antiquated and does not have fields to enter nonbinary gender identities or name preferences and you also note many discrepancies in pronoun use and documentation of gender identity in provider notes. You notice that the resident called the patient "Mr. R" during your return call, and wonder whether this is an unintentional error or reflects a personal choice of the patient.

Your chart review further reveals a history of high emergency room utilization, frequent admissions for respiratory and gastrointestinal infections, and visits related to intoxication from alcohol, cocaine, methamphetamine, and opioids. There are scattered visits for sexually transmitted infection (STI) testing and treatment. Many of these notes document concurrent nonadherence to ART. During the present admission, you see that the patient's failure to thrive was initially felt to be related to oropharyngeal candidiasis with alteration in taste and odynophagia. The patient's CD4 count on admission was found to be 240 cells/mm^3 with a viral load of 11,000 copies/mL. Antifungal treatment was initiated and ART was restarted. Notes show that oral discomfort has resolved and the team is uncertain why the patient's nutritional intake has not improved. You attempt to call the primary resident back to clarify details about the team's concern for an underlying psychiatric illness as well as the patient's gender identity but there is no answer.

On your way to the patient's room, one of the unit nurses stops you and expresses relief that psychiatry has been called to see this patient, as the nurses all feel there must be something "psychiatrically wrong…a personality disorder or something" to explain the patient's rude treatment of staff and unpredictable mood. The nurse reports that the patient frequently voices derogatory and dismissive retorts to nursing and nursing support staff when food trays and medications are brought in as if the attentive care they are providing is aversive.

Before entering the patient's room, you remind yourself to inquire about what name and pronouns this patient uses. In introductions, you learn that Ms. R has socially transitioned, uses a typically feminine name and prefers the feminine pronouns she/her/hers. Ms. R also has a stereotypically feminine gender expression with long curled hair, painted nails, hoop earrings, and heavily applied makeup. Though you wonder if she has undergone gender-affirming medical and/or surgical treatment, you defer asking any questions on this topic that are not immediately relevant to the consultation until you have established rapport and provided a safe therapeutic space [13].

Ms. R quickly expresses appreciation at your having inquired about her name instead of using the name assigned at birth and on her legal documents and medical record. She immediately launches into many complaints about mistreatment by her medical providers and others in her life. She adds that she does not trust doctors because they have never proved themselves to be trustworthy, "you doctors are more interested in my genitals than my health and make me feel like a total freak show!" You validate her experiences and begin to internally connect Ms. R's anger and mistrust of authority with the team's perception that she is hostile and rejecting. When you explain that you have been consulted because the team is worried about her refusal of food and medications, you ask whether these behaviors are related to mistrust or feeling mistreated. She snidely replies, "So they assume I'm crazy because I won't go along with protocol? Those robotic doctors are the real lunatics."

You elicit a full psychiatric and social history from Ms. R while being aware of any assumptions you might be making in your countertransference and emphasizing the use of inclusive and affirming language for sexual and gender minority people. You learn that Ms. R has never seen a psychiatrist outside of psychiatric assessments in the emergency room when she is either agitated or intoxicated. She has chosen not to follow up with referrals made during these encounters explaining that mental illness was always stigmatized in her predominantly Catholic, Puerto Rican family. Her family disowned her during late adolescence when she began to take steps to affirm and align her gender expression with her gender identity by asking others to use female pronouns and call her by a feminine name and to accept her dressing as a girl. She did not complete high school and has frequently been fired from jobs due to discrimination related to her transgender identity or her difficulties with emotion regulation. She supports herself through sex work and is homeless, primarily sleeping on couches, the street, or sporadically in shelters. Ms. R began to use illicit substances during childhood as a means to regulate her mood and to escape her reality, a wish stemming both from internalized transphobia and the real dangers of living as a trans person. She has recently been using marijuana and cocaine regularly "to forget all of the traumatic stuff that has happened to me."

When you inquire more about her history of trauma, Ms. R lists multiple instances of sexual assault that occurred in her line of sex work, as well as intimate partner violence in two prior romantic relationships. She mentions a physical assault, which occurred on the subway and quickly rushes past her early life, noting the "unending horror of it all." You tactfully request clarification, and she describes instances of sexual molestation by an older sibling. Symptomatically Ms. R meets DSM 5 diagnostic criteria [3] for Post-Traumatic Stress Disorder (PTSD) related to these traumatic experiences, in addition to comorbid recurrent major depressive disorder and multiple substance use disorders. You note again that her substance use functions in part as a means of avoidance, regulating symptoms of hyper-arousal and intrusion.

At the end of the interview, you return to an exploration of Ms. R's mistrust of doctors and figures of authority and inquire whether this accounts for her not taking ART or engaging in outpatient medical care. She agrees with the interpretation and states that since her body has only brought her pain and suffering it warrants such neglect. You spend time educating Ms. R about PTSD, and describe how the establishment of trust and social attachments is often impaired in victims of early-life physical, sexual, and emotional abuse, especially when perpetrated by family members.

Ms. R responds positively to learning about the diagnostic criteria for PTSD and availability of evidence-based psychotherapeutic treatment to which she is more open than medication. You provide an overview of therapy modalities including Prolonged Exposure (PE), Cognitive Processing Therapy (CPT), and Trauma-Focused Cognitive Behavioral Therapy (TF-CBT), which directly address memories of the traumatic events or maladaptive thoughts and feelings related to the trauma [14]. You suggest to her that the avoidance seen in PTSD as well as associated shame and guilt are all factors contributing to her nonadherence to ART. Together you brainstorm about ways in which she might communicate more effectively with hospital support staff and treatment providers to ensure that her needs are met in respectful and safe therapeutic relationships. You find yourself thinking that the quality of the clinical encounter is not Ms. R's responsibility alone to ensure; providers who hope to reach the most vulnerable might begin by asking and using their preferred name.

You return to the team to share your impression that Ms. R is suffering from PTSD and that her food and medication refusal is most likely an angry rejection of anything provided by an authority figure to protect herself from feeling out of control, vulnerable, and helpless in a medical setting. You provide them with outpatient options for individual and group therapy modalities. You recommend that they refer Ms. R to an integrated HIV care center where awareness of the specific needs of the lesbian, gay, bisexual, transgender, and queer (LGBTQ) community will inform health care, thus mitigating the discrimination the patient may have experienced in the past. The team expresses appreciation for your recommendation and plans to facilitate the referral.

You offer brief education to the resident about the higher incidence of traumatic experiences in transgender people and also in persons living with HIV [11, 15]. You refer to the history of discrimination that these individuals historically have faced within health-care settings. You explain the importance of using the pronouns preferred by the patient as a core validation of their personhood and as a fundamental basis for establishing trust in the clinical encounter. You also provide a medical explanation for HPA (hypothalamic-pituitary-adrenal) axis dysfunction, which occurs when individuals are exposed to violence, sexual abuse, and adverse childhood experiences, describing how this may impair regulation, attention, and hyper-vigilance leading to difficulties in self-care and care for others [16, 17]. The resident responds by explaining that he has not received training on best practices for the culturally competent care of transgender patients and expresses interest in learning more. He asks if he might facilitate an in-service with the psychiatry consult service to provide education on trauma-informed care and an affirming approach to working with transgender patients. You wholeheartedly accept this invitation, you thank the resident for allowing you to advocate on the patient's behalf, and you reflect on the underlying courage and resilience of so many within the trans population.

Appendix: Summary Table

	Problems	Strategies
• Patient symptoms and behaviors	• Depression: negative self-appraisal and cognitions leading to refusal of care and nutrition, suicidal ideation • Neurocognitive: Memory impairment, functional impairment • Psychosis: Delusions, hallucinations, disordered thought process • Trauma: post-traumatic stress disorder (PTSD) symptoms interfering with self-care, mood regulation, and social relationships	• Guide diagnostic clarification, provide treatment recommendations that address any comorbidities, and facilitate ongoing psychiatric care • Assist in clarifying manifestations of psychiatric illness versus HIV-associated neurocognitive disorders • Advocate for discharge plan that addresses patient's functional needs and quality of life • Provide safe recommendations for use of neuroleptics when indicated • Educate the patient and team on symptoms associated with trauma and PTSD and their impact on self-care • Motivate and engage the patient for longer-term follow-up and adherence to medical and mental health treatment
• Provider-patient dynamics	• Provider feels ineffective and helpless in the face of complex longitudinal patient care needs and barriers in accessing resources. May lead to defensive appraisal of patient behaviors as volitional and a desire to "be rid" of the patient from their service • Dynamics of patient anger and hostile behaviors coupled with defensive team behaviors to avoid anxiety and feelings of ineffectiveness related to limitations in knowledge about transgender and trauma informed care	• Validate reality-based frustrations in systems of care and educate on bio-psycho-social burden of comorbid severe and persistent mental illness, substance use, and HIV • Advocate for the patient's wishes. Consider additional team members who may provide helpful expertise and support • Normalize and humanize the patient's behaviors as part of their history of trauma and experiences of discrimination in the healthcare setting. Address gaps in provider knowledge with compassion

• Patient-provider barriers	• Patient mistrust and hostile engagement related to experiences of stigma and discrimination by healthcare professionals	• Validate the patient's experiences and assist in brainstorming concrete ways to improve communication to get patient needs met • Educate the team as needed to help facilitate safe and respectful interactions with the patient
• Hospital system barriers	• Patient requires a higher level of care upon discharge from hospital and comorbid psychiatric and/or substance use disorders complicate the process	• Consider additional diagnostic evaluation to support the need for a higher level of care • Consider additional resources including inter-professional and other social supports who may be resources for the team to help facilitate a safe discharge from the hospital

References

1. Reda AA. Edited by Alex Mitchell. Reliability and validity of the Ethiopian version of the hospital anxiety and depression scale (HADS) in HIV infected patients. PloS One. 2001;6(1):e16049.
2. Zhan W. Depressive symptoms and unprotected sex in St. Petersburg, Russia. J Psychosom Res. 2012;72(5):371–5.
3. American Psychiatric Association. Diagnostic and statistical manual of mental disorders. 5th ed. Washington, DC: American Psychiatric Association; 2013.
4. Grov C. Loneliness and HIV-related stigma explain depression among older HIV-positive adults. AIDS Care. 2010;22(5):630–9.
5. Wagner GJ. A closer look at depression and its relationship to HIV antiretroviral adherence. Ann Behav Med. 2011;42(3):352–60.
6. Finlay L. Relational integrative psychotherapy: process and theory in practice. Chichester: Wiley; 2015.
7. Bagashev A, Sawaya B. Roles and functions of HIV-1 tat protein in the CNS: an overview. Virol J. 2013;10:358.
8. Wellbutrin. Physicians' desk reference. 67th ed. Montvale, NJ: PDR Network; 2013.
9. Modafanil. Physicians' desk reference. 67th ed. Montvale, NJ: PDR Network; 2013.
10. Francisco C. HIV-related movement disorders. CNS Drugs. 2002;16:663–8.
11. LeGrand S. A review of recent literature on trauma among individuals living with HIV. Curr HIV/AIDS Rep. 2015;12(4):397–405.
12. Yehia BR. Barriers and facilitators to patient retention in HIV care. BMC Infect Dis. 2015;15:246.
13. Yarbrough E. Transgender mental health. 1st ed. Washington, DC: American Psychiatric Association; 2018.
14. Watts BV. Meta-analysis of the efficacy of treatments for posttraumatic stress disorder. J Clin Psychiatry. 2013;74(6):e541–50.
15. Beckman K. Military sexual assault in transgender veterans: results from a Nationwide study. J Trauma Stress. 2018;31(2):181–90.
16. Felitti VJ, Anda RF, Nordenberg D, Edwards V, Koss MP, Marks JS. Relationship of childhood abuse and household dysfunction to many causes of death in adults: the adverse childhood experiences (ACE) study. J Prev Med. 1998;14(4):245–58.
17. Neigh GN, Gillespie C, Nemeroff CB. The neurobiological toll of child abuse and neglect. Trauma Violence Abuse. 2009;10(4):389–410.

Further Reading

Citron K, Brouillette MJ, Beckett A. HIV and psychiatry: a training and resource manual. 2nd ed. Cambridge: Cambridge University Press; 2005.

Cohen MA, Gorman JM, Jacobson JM, Volberding P, Letendre SL. Comprehensive textbook of AIDS psychiatry: a paradigm for integrated care. 2nd ed. New York: Oxford University Press; 2017. Chapters 6, 9, 11, 12, 15-17, 19, 41, 42, 50.

Levenson J. The American Psychiatric Association Publishing textbook of psychosomatic medicine and consultation-liaison psychiatry. Washington, DC: American Psychiatric Association; 2019. Chapters 26 and 39.

The Postpartum Patient

6

Alyson Gorun and Alison Hermann

Your pager reads: "Ms. P is saying odd things about her newborn, can you assess her?"

Psychiatric symptoms in postpartum patients can generate significant anxiety for the primary medical or obstetrics team. This page is asking—has there been a change in the patient's mental status? If so, could it be due to an underlying psychiatric disorder, or psychiatric symptoms emerging in the postpartum period? Diagnostically, the word "odd" may imply a thought disorder with pathological thought content related to the newborn (e.g., delusions or obsessions). It may also imply a broad range of other diagnoses in addition to unique risks associated with the postpartum period, including substance intoxication or withdrawal, delirium, personality disorders, obsessive-compulsive disorder, mood disorders, an attachment disorder, or other diagnostic categories. While all of these diagnoses are important for the health and wellness of this new mother, the primary diagnosis of concern as the psychiatric consultant immediately postpartum is psychosis. This

A. Gorun (✉)
Weill Cornell Medicine, New York-Presbyterian Hospital,
New York, NY, USA

A. Hermann
Department of Psychiatry, NewYork-Presbyterian Hospital/
Weill Cornell Medicine, New York, NY, USA
e-mail: alh9039@med.cornell.edu

A. Gorun et al. (eds.), *The Psychiatric Consult*,
https://doi.org/10.1007/978-3-031-26837-3_6

is a psychiatric emergency that typically requires inpatient psychiatric hospitalization to ensure the safety of the patient and her infant [1]. Clarifying what the team means by "odd" will be important since many nonpsychiatric providers can use this or similarly vague words as a nonspecific catch-all for behavioral or thought disturbances, without awareness of the implications on what might be occurring diagnostically.

The essential question the team may be asking is if Ms. P is safe to go home with her newborn, able to appropriately care for her newborn outside of the hospital, and ultimately if the team (or psychiatry) needs to intervene to maintain both mother and infant safety. The safety assessment for a postpartum consultation involves an evaluation of the infant's safety risk in addition to the mother's, including the risk of the mother harming herself or her infant, as well as the mother's ability to meet the infant's basic needs within the context of possible psychiatric symptoms.

The relationship between mothers and infants forms the basis of adult relationships and therefore providers caring for mother-infant dyads are particularly vulnerable to experiencing subtle and yet powerful countertransference reactions [2]. Strong provider-patient countertransference reactions may also occur toward mothers with psychiatric illness specifically, including anxious, fearful, or frustrated feelings generated from a provider's own experience of their parents or being a parent themselves. Questions from the team regarding the need for psychiatric hospitalization or withholding or initiating psychotropic treatment may be a reactive or appropriate response to fears regarding the safety of the newborn, and the potentially grave consequences of inadequately treated postpartum psychosis or severe depression. An awareness of these dynamics is critical to enabling optimal safety and treatment planning, while avoiding over- or undertreatment of these patients.

Clinical Scenario

You review the chart and read that Ms. P is a 28-year-old woman, gravida 1 and para 1 (G1P1) woman who had a normal spontaneous vaginal delivery 1 day ago. You call the obstetrics and gynecology (OB/GYN) resident to get more information. The resident tells you that a nurse had informed her that Ms. P had been saying "odd" things about her newborn that morning, and urged her to consult psychiatry to assess the patient. You attempt to clarify the nature of Ms. P's comments by asking for more details about what Ms. P said and whether there were any associated behaviors of concern. The resident says she saw the patient this morning and that she seemed "very anxious" but she didn't note anything "odd" about Ms. P's presentation. She does tell you that Ms. P seemed to have trouble understanding some of the preparatory instructions for discharge, but she thought it may have just been because she was feeling overwhelmed in her role as a new mother.

Scenario 1: Bipolar Disorder and Pregnancy

You ask the OB/GYN resident for more of Ms. P's psychiatric history. The resident says she tried to gather more information for the consult but found Ms. P's answers to be "vague and confusing." The resident says Ms. P did allude to having a psychiatric history, but wasn't able to clarify.

As you prepare to see Ms. P you notice a feeling of frustration with the resident that she had not gotten some of the basic information you'd want before seeing Ms. P. After knocking on Ms. P's door and introducing yourself as a psychiatric consultant, you take note when you entered that she is dressed in her street clothes, writing in a notebook, and that her new baby is in a bassinet at her bedside. Ms. P immediately puts the notebook away and tells you that she was told that you would be coming to speak to her "just to check in" before she is discharged home. You ask her how she is feeling after the delivery but instead of answering your question she immediately tells you she has an outpatient psychiatrist whom she hasn't seen in many months. She then begins to tangentially describe various seemingly unrelated events from her past. You note that Ms. P is speaking very quickly, is pressured, and is difficult to interrupt. Although you initially feel that you're able to effortfully follow what she's saying, you realize after being in the room with her for 20 minutes you continue to have little understanding of her psychiatric history. When you attempt to narrow your questions and clarify some of the basic information without success, you find yourself feeling again frustrated and now confused by how challenging it has been to obtain the information you'll need to make an assessment. You wonder to yourself if the feeling of confusion that you are experiencing is similar to the feeling of confusion the OB/GYN resident experienced when attempting to communicate with Ms. P. You start to recognize that the difficulty multiple health-care providers have had communicating with Ms. P may be an indication that Ms. P is displaying symptoms of a thought disorder. Given the patient's pressured speech and likely flight of ideas, you are worried she may be experiencing symptoms of a bipolar spectrum disorder, and ask the patient for consent to speak to her outpatient psychiatrist to get more collateral information, which she agrees to.

Although it is difficult to conduct the interview, requiring you to redirect Ms. P multiple times, you pursue a critical safety evaluation, focusing your questions to those pertinent to Ms. P and to the newborn's safety with Ms. P outside of the monitored setting of the hospital. Ms. P says she is planning on returning home alone with her newborn for the next several days before the father of the baby—who she is planning to co-parent with—will be returning to share childcare responsibilities. She says she hadn't planned to see her psychiatrist in the postpartum period, despite her psychiatrist instructing her to call him after she gave birth, because she had been feeling "the best I've felt in my entire life," and didn't think there was a reason to follow up. Nothing Ms. P said was illogical or bizarre, but there were several aspects of her presentation that were unusual for a woman who was immediately postpartum, including indications of an abnormally elevated mood and thought disorganization more severe than could be explained by anxiety. Additionally, there is a lack of a plan for support during the immediate postpartum period, including a denial of the difficulties of neonatal care and potential risks postpartum for someone with a history of psychiatric symptoms. You ask about any intrusive thoughts to hurt the baby or herself and she responds with surprise, "of course not!". She then pulls out multiple additional notebooks she had hidden underneath her bed and starts to show you what she has written inside saying, "See, I'm taking very good care of him." She begins going through disorganized notes tracking every behavior and movement the new baby has made as well as which doctors and nurses have come in and out of her room. Some of the notes say "Is there something wrong with the baby? Did Nurse X put something in my milk? Is the milk contaminated?" You ask about this note, asking her if she is concerned about the baby's health. She says "Well, yes, no… I'm not sure," then looks around the room furtively and takes the notebook away from you. She then asks for your name and credentials and says she'd like to be discharged soon. You let her know you need to speak to her outpatient psychiatrist first. At this point you are very concerned that Ms. P is paranoid and you immediately let the OB/GYN resident know that she cannot be discharged until you complete your evaluation and recommend a one-to-one for elopement precautions.

When you call her outpatient psychiatrist, you discover that she experienced a manic episode a few years ago that required psychiatric hospitalization and was marked by paranoia that resulted in her not eating and severe weight loss. She was treated with lithium at that time and had remained on lithium up until she found out that she was pregnant, at which point she discontinued the medication. You become increasingly concerned that Ms. P is displaying symptoms of a postpartum manic episode with psychotic features, and that she has no treatment plan for when she returns home. A comprehensive strategy to reduce maternal and infant risk postpartum for women with mood disorders should include symptom monitoring (e.g., significant changes in behavior that may be indicative of mania or psychosis) by the patient and identified support system, interventions to protect sleep and minimize stress, and a planned follow-up visit with their mental health provider, among others [3]. As you formulate your recommendation for an appropriate disposition for Ms. P, you consider that you are concerned about her and her infant's safety, and also are aware of how painful the process of separating from her infant for the hospitalization may be. You remind yourself internally of the known safety risks associated with inadequately treated and monitored postpartum psychosis, including more prominent cognitive deficits such as disorientation and confusion (and the resulting potential for neglect), as well as infanticide and suicide [1]. The delusional content involving her infant is particularly concerning given its new onset and the uncertainty in how this will affect the infant's care at home. You discuss your clinical reasoning with your attending, who validates your concerns about safety, and you both agree she requires psychiatric hospitalization, despite anticipating the patient's anger and distress at being separated from her child. You are surprised that when you speak to the patient about her symptoms and the recommendation for hospitalization, she agrees that maybe she isn't "feeling quite like [herself]," could benefit from "sleep and some time to recover" in the hospital, and that "maybe the baby will be safer with his father." You facilitate her contacting the father of the baby to arrange for him to take care of him while she is in the hospital.

There isn't immediate bed availability on an inpatient psychiatric unit, so you inform the OB/GYN resident that Ms. P will need to stay on their floor until a bed becomes available. The resident asks you for medication recommendations. You remember Ms. P was able to tell you that she would like to continue breastfeeding, and you initially decide to recommend quetiapine after a review of its safety data related to breastfeeding on LactMed [4]. The resident calls you and says Ms. P doesn't want to take any psychiatric medication, because she doesn't want to hurt her baby. The resident expresses frustration to you that Ms. P is "refusing to accept treatment" even though she is clearly symptomatic. She also expresses her belief that this will prolong her hospitalization and separation from her newborn. She says to you, "she should've never stopped taking her medication." You pause and take note of the resident's frustration and wonder to yourself what might be behind it. You reflect that there could be multiple coexisting etiologies, including the resident's own need to be a "good" doctor, a desire to complete her workload and go home, or an ambition to fulfill the expectations of her superiors. She may also be responding to the difficulty of witnessing an incapacitated mother be separated from her baby or to her own wish to be the surrogate decision-maker for Ms. P.

You decide to discuss with the OB/GYN resident the need to preserve Ms. P's autonomy as much as possible when discussing the medication options, reframing the conversation to center around Ms. P's needs at the moment. You take time to help the resident process that Ms. P is indeed motivated by the desire to be a good mother and to protect her baby, and is not motivated by a desire to frustrate the team or complicate her treatment. You tell the resident that you'll outline for her the risks of exposure to the recommended medications while breastfeeding as well as the risks of untreated bipolar disorder in the postpartum period to the baby and herself to see if you can address Ms. P's concerns. When you meet with Ms. P again, you encourage her to have a trusted support person present to help her with her decision-making, who can not only assist the patient in decision-making while having manic and psychotic symptoms, but can also assist in monitoring of symptoms and medication adherence when Ms. P returns home. After an extensive discussion, Ms. P ultimately decides that she does want to take quetiapine, and thanks you.

In this scenario, Ms. P is experiencing a postpartum manic episode with psychotic features. Women with bipolar disorder are at high risk for relapse of mood symptoms in the postpartum period [5]. For a woman who is already taking lithium like Ms. P, lithium discontinuation itself may be a risk factor for the recurrence of mood symptoms [6]. Known risks of lithium use during pregnancy include a small potential increase in the risk for cardiac malformations including Ebstein's anomaly; however, this risk is much lower than previously described. Otherwise, there appears to be no other increased risk of malformations, and limited data shows no effect on obstetric or neurodevelopmental outcomes. Taken together, this means that pregnancy and breastfeeding are no longer considered absolute contraindications for the use of lithium in women with bipolar disorder. Stratifying the risk of illness relapse for a mother include considerations such as the severity of illness (e.g., frequency and severity of episodes, number of hospitalizations, age of illness onset), risk behaviors associated with illness (e.g., violence, suicide attempts, self-neglect including lack of treatment engagement or medical nonadherence), substance use history, and level of social support. It is essential to weigh the risks of lithium use against the risks of untreated bipolar disorder to both the mother and the developing fetus when determining optimal treatment [3].

A clinician may unwittingly attempt to assume a parental role as decision-maker if there is a difference in the clinician's recommendations and mother's choice about medication use or other aspects of her treatment. This can be exacerbated and become problematic if there is underlying provider anxiety about the fetus or infant's safety despite an objective lack of safety concerns. Provider anxiety could be driven by a number of underlying factors such as a fear of liability in cases of fetal or infant harm, or by a clinician's anxious countertransference driven by an overidentification with the mother or infant, a need to control or please others, or other unconscious factors. The mother's choices may be based on underlying values, cultural norms, or prior experiences with medications or psychiatric treatment, and should be incorporated into treatment decisions. Overly parental or authoritative recommendations can potentially lead to disregard of the mother's needs and perspectives. Shared decision-making including a careful risk-benefit analysis and collaborative treatment and safety planning is a crucial way to protect a mother's autonomy.

Scenario 2: Postpartum Psychosis

By the time you see Ms. P, she is pacing around her room and yelling loudly that someone has been trying to poison her and her newborn and she needs help. You attempt to verbally de-escalate the situation by reflecting back Ms. P's concerns in an effort to contain her affect. You say, "someone is trying to poison you?" She stops pacing and looks at you intensely and repeats "yes and no one is doing anything about it!" You gently ask her how does she know she has been poisoned. She says she knows because she has a headache and feels "tingly" and numb throughout the left side of her body. She wants to see a "real" doctor immediately and then yells at you to "get out." Since the patient is agitated and refuses to engage in a psychiatric interview, you leave the room. As you leave the unit, Ms. P's husband approaches you in the waiting room. He tells you that the patient has never behaved like this before, and her presentation is a shock to him. He tells you quietly that she told him that she thinks she's being infected by a poison and had attempted to scratch her arms to get the poison out. You reflect back that it sounds like this is very unlike her, and he says yes, she was completely herself up until the birth. He doesn't think it's psychiatric because as far as he knows she's never had any psychiatric issues in the past. You ask if she's ever had any issues with any drugs or alcohol, and he says "no, never! She really has never had any issues before this."

Although you are not sure whether the physical symptoms she disclosed to you have a nonpsychiatric etiology, you see that there has been no medical workup done in the chart and no mention of her headache or unilateral numbness. You recommend to the OB/GYN resident obtaining a medical workup of the patient's symptoms to rule out any nonpsychiatric causes of her physical symptoms and her psychosis, in addition to a neurology consult. You internally reframe the differential to include common conditions which may cause altered mental status during the postpartum period including autoimmune diseases or an infectious process [1]. Given her vague neurological symptoms, it would be important to have an objective neurologic exam that can assess for overt motor symptoms or dyskinesias and investigate whether her symptoms were stemming from a neurological disease. Her neurological symptoms might indicate an increased chance of anti-N-methyl-D-aspartate receptor (NMDAR) encephalitis, which has been described as a specific concern in the postpartum period, and prompt further workup [1]. You also let the resident know that Ms. P had scratched herself because of a delusion and recommend one-to-one observation of the patient due to her risk of self-harm and agitation as well as provide recommendations for medications for acute agitation if needed. If Ms. P is medically cleared you let the resident know she will require inpatient psychiatric hospitalization.

That afternoon, you receive a follow up call from the OB/GYN resident, who informs you that Ms. P already appears "better" and is no longer saying anything that strikes the team as "odd." The resident says she has been interacting appropriately with her family and staff members—in fact, her husband says that she's returned to her baseline and seems back to normal. The neurology consultant obtained additional history that Ms. P has chronic headaches of similar quality and her neurologic exam did not have any abnormal focal findings. All of Ms. P's vital signs, blood work (including thyroid studies and an ammonia level), magnetic resonance imaging of her brain, urinalysis, and urine toxicology were also without any abnormal findings. Given her report of neurologic symptoms with new onset of psychosis, the consultant conducted a lumbar puncture and did not find any evidence of anti-NMDAR encephalitis in Ms. P's cerebrospinal fluid analysis. Serum antibodies are a less invasive screening tool; however, they are frequently falsely positive making this a less useful clinical tool. They have signed off without recommending further intervention. You cross reference the medical workup suggested for postpartum psychosis [1] and note that everything pertinent in this population has been ruled out.

The resident asks you if Ms. P really needs psychiatric admission since it seems like she has already improved and her family at bedside doesn't want her to be separated from her newborn or admitted to a psychiatric hospital. The resident mentions that she is a mother herself and knows how hard it can be to be away from her own children. You take note of the resident's response—one of empathy, but also of potential overidentification with Ms. P, a process which may unconsciously and subtly influence her perspective on the recommended treatment. You provide psychoeducation to the resident regarding the waxing and waning presentation of postpartum psychosis that may contribute to the perception that Ms. P is "better." You also explain the associated elevated risk for infanticide and suicide, and the details of your safety assessment. After clearly explaining the clinical decision-making and necessary considerations of safety in this high-risk population, the resident seems less anxious about your recommendation and agrees that the patient needs psychiatric hospitalization.

When you go to Ms. P's room to speak to her family about psychiatric hospitalization, one of Ms. P's brothers introduces himself as someone with experience in the medical field and states firmly that "this is not a psychiatric issue, but a medical one" and requests that additional medical consultations and bloodwork be ordered. He elaborates that he researched Ms. P's symptoms and thinks that she has anti-NMDAR encephalitis—he tells you she should be seen by the neurologist again and does not understand why a psychiatrist is involved. You ask for Ms. P's brother to briefly step out of the room in order to ask Ms. P for consent to speak to him, which she agrees to. You then pause to consider what may be the underlying motivation behind her brother's concerns as you bring him back into the room with Ms. P, and then share with her and her brother that she has already been seen by neurology and assessed appropriately for this condition, though you avoid going into details because you're not sure whether you're prepared to answer all of his questions about the neurologic workup. He replies that he doesn't want her labeled a "psych patient" before everything "medical" has been ruled out sufficiently. You acknowledge the brother's concerns, and share that a psychiatric hospitalization is a medical hospitalization, and a way to continue to monitor and treat Ms. P's symptoms, and that appropriate medical interventions can occur should her symptoms change or worsen. You notice yourself becoming very uncomfortable and somewhat defensive as you did not expect and feel unprepared for a conflict with Ms. P's brother. In an attempt to partner with him and diffuse conflict, you decide to reframe her symptoms using a medical model of disease by describing the rapid shift in estrogen and progesterone after giving birth that may contribute to an increased risk of symptoms, in general, postpartum. The possible role of genetics, postpartum activation of the immune system, and circadian rhythm changes, are also discussed as potential factors in the etiology of psychiatric symptoms postpartum. At this point, you shift the conversation toward Ms. P's safety rather than giving a psychiatric diagnosis, and avoid using the term "postpartum psychosis" as well as any firm impression that her symptoms are psychiatric, since safety seems to be the shared goal between you and the family and you hope will increase acceptance of the recommendation for a psychiatric hospitalization. The family is able to agree with this, especially after Ms. P's husband contributes the information regarding how Ms. P believed she had been poisoned so had scratched her arms to get it out. Ms.

P vocalizes concerns about being able to see her newborn while in the hospital and continuing to breastfeed. You confirm that she will be able to pump while hospitalized, and discuss the procedures for visitation while there. At the end of the discussion, Ms. P and her brother continue to believe that she is not psychiatrically ill but they agree that she does need to continue to be monitored in a hospital setting, and ultimately consent to the transfer, with your reassurances.

A couple of days later you receive a phone call from your coresident who took over care of Ms. P on the inpatient psychiatric unit. She tells you that since Ms. P arrived, the family and patient have been insistent that she needs further medical workup including multiple requests to reconsult neurology and for additional invasive medical workup. She reached out to you to ask whether you thought there was a possibility that her symptoms were consistent with anti-NMDAR encephalitis or another nonpsychiatric disease process, even though the lumbar puncture was negative. She comments that it's been extremely challenging to maintain a tenuous rapport with the family and Ms. P. You note that this is the same interaction you had with the family previously, and realize that you did not discuss your specific diagnostic impressions or explain why further medical workup was not indicated, putting your coresident in the same position that you were in. You think about your own anxiety in talking to the family that led to an avoidance of an appropriate dialogue about her psychiatric symptoms, including feeling intimidated and possibly unable to contain the family's fears about a potentially stigmatizing diagnosis and associated genetic implications if Ms. P desired more biologic children.

You decide to disclose to your coresident how uncomfortable you felt interacting with Ms. P and her brother and your decision to diffuse the situation via medicalization of Ms. P's illness. You now think there might have been other motivators, including an identification with Ms. P or her distressed family member that discouraged a full and direct discussion of her psychiatric diagnosis. You tell your coresident your avoidance of the discussion could reflect Ms. P and her family's own avoidance of the fear and anxieties associated with a psychiatric diagnosis. You suggest they have a family meeting to review her medical workup, including the recommendations regarding assessment for anti-NMDAR receptor encephalitis [7], and creating a space for Ms. P to openly discuss her anxieties and fears about her diagnosis and hospital course.

In this scenario, both the clinicians and family members are having difficulty with the diagnosis of postpartum psychosis for a new mother. Strong countertransference reactions can potentially be precipitated by the presence of the newborn—the OB/GYN resident seems to partially overidentify with the mother, something that early-career clinicians may be more vulnerable to given they may be new parents themselves or similar in age. Additionally, early-career clinicians may not have had enough experience to see first-hand how dangerous and unpredictable psychosis in the postpartum period can be if left untreated, as well as being falsely reassured by the periods of clarity during which they interact with a patient, not realizing that the patient's symptoms may be waxing and waning. This can potentially lead to a minimizing of symptoms and undertreatment of a patient. Within families, a desire to "protect" the patient and themselves from the loss of a previously healthy family member, as well as stigma associated with psychiatric diagnoses, can lead to a refusal of psychiatric involvement or to over-involvement of unnecessary medical consultations and workup (each of which can carry risks of their own). Given the rapid and dramatic onset of symptoms associated with postpartum psychosis, especially in cases with no prior history, medical and/or neurologic explanations may seem more plausible to patients and their families than psychiatric explanations. If the psychiatric consultant is not able to adequately address these assumptions, then putting forward a psychiatric diagnosis may lead to powerful fears of misdiagnosis and medical neglect in the patient and her family. This could increase conflict in their relationship with the team of primary providers.

Emphasizing the medical nature of a psychiatric hospitalization and treatment, including the potential hormonal influence on precipitating current symptoms, can make psychiatric treatment initially more acceptable for a family and patient struggling to cope with such a change. However, it is also important to recognize that the avoidance of an appropriate diagnostic and treatment discussion, including only emphasizing the “medical” nature of a patient’s symptoms, may be a response to the family and patient’s own fears about the diagnosis. Being able to accurately read the emotional underpinnings and motivation behind a family and patient’s engagement and requests, validating and containing them, and maintaining an evidence-based management despite conflicting emotional cues, is necessary when managing these patients.

Ms. P expressed appropriate concern regarding the separation of herself from her infant via psychiatric hospitalization. There is an increasing number of mother-baby inpatient psychiatric units and other care settings in the United States, but the demand far outweighs the availability, and these units exists in few areas of the United States [8]. Acknowledging the impact of separating mother and baby, and attempting to address their concerns by arranging for supplies for pumping and appropriately supervised mother–infant interaction on the unit (once determined to be safe) can help mitigate this, and facilitate the necessary treatment.

Scenario 3: Postpartum Depression

When you arrive at Ms. P’s room, you notice that she is holding her new baby but appears uncomfortable, tentative and unsure of herself while moving him around. After you introduce yourself and your role, Ms. P tells you that she has been feeling increasingly depressed and anxious, a change that began in the third trimester. At time of onset, she had difficulty sleeping despite having the opportunity to sleep and was awake all night worrying about something bad happening to the baby or herself. She was quick to dismiss this, noting that she thought difficulty sleeping was normal for women who are pregnant. She goes on to say that she thinks not sleeping has made it more difficult for her to make even the smallest decisions about planning for the postpartum period, and that she has been afraid of making a choice that could potentially negatively affect her baby. You tell her, “I can see how important it is to you to do a good job caring for your baby,” and she smiles reluctantly. You register her somewhat flat response, and comment that sometimes a symptom of depression is difficulty bonding with a newborn and ask her if this is something she has been experiencing. She tells you softly, yes, that she feels like she should be having warmer feelings toward him—in fact she has felt detached from him. She begins crying and tells you that she wishes she could be "replaced with a different mother who could be better than [her]" and thinks maybe the baby would be better off without a mother who can't love him.

You follow up with more questions about these statements, revealing that she has been thinking that it would be easier to maybe not be alive and that she has a desire to fall asleep and not wake up. She then cuts you off to emphasize that she would never try to hurt herself, citing her new baby as a protective factor. You keep in mind that postpartum depression frequently presents with anxiety, specifically about the baby or the baby's health. Obsessive thoughts regarding a mother harming her baby that are intrusive, unwanted, and not consistent with a mother's desires are also common and can be particularly shameful and difficult for a mother to disclose—not only because they are afraid of acting on them, but also because she may be aware that clinicians can and sometimes do misinterpret these thoughts as being ego-syntonic and associated with increased risk [9]. Explicitly asking about intrusive thoughts and normalizing them can help a mother be more open about her symptoms. You ask Ms. P if she's experienced any unwanted intrusive thoughts to harm her baby, including thoughts such as stabbing or drowning the baby, or odd things such as putting the baby in a microwave. You explain that these are common in general for women in the postpartum period, as well as in women with postpartum depression, and does not mean that she would like to do these things or that there is a risk that she would actually act on them [10]. She says "Thank goodness I don't have any of those!", and adds that this is the first time she's ever had thoughts of not wanting to be alive and has never tried to act on those thoughts. You ask her if she's ever been depressed in the past or if she's ever taken any medication for depression, and she replies that she had been depressed before but that it never felt as bad as it did now. She says she was first diagnosed with depression many years ago and started escitalopram, a serotonin reuptake inhibitor (SSRI), and that this helped get rid of her depression. She stayed on this up until she found out she was pregnant and at that time stopped taking it. For the first few months after stopping it she felt "okay." When you ask her about her decision-making around stopping escitalopram, she said she didn't want to be taking anything that could potentially harm her pregnancy. When she started to notice feeling depressed and anxious a few months ago she returned to therapy, joined a support group, and started working on stress management techniques. Unfortunately, they didn't alleviate her symptoms.

Although you feel confident that Ms. P's symptoms are consistent with postpartum depression, you decide to administer an Edinburgh Postnatal Depression Scale (EPDS) to characterize the severity and as a data point when you discuss the risks of depression and anxiety with Ms. P. The EPDS accounts for depression and anxiety as well as normal physiologic changes that occur during pregnancy, making it a particularly useful tool for the postpartum patient. She scores 15, which indicates a moderate depression [11] and you share this information with Ms. P. She says, "wow, I didn't realize I was feeling so badly." You reflect that it does seem that she has been suffering and ask about her thoughts on restarting her escitalopram. She appears tense and says that she knows she's depressed but that she wanted to breastfeed. She tells you, "I'm already constantly worried about things that could harm him, I can't bear to add more things to worry about. I would feel so guilty if something bad happened to him just because I wanted to feel better." You note your own feeling of obligation to treat Ms. P's depression and be an effective resident, and how this quickly makes you want to convince her that taking escitalopram while breastfeeding is "100% safe." However, you take a step back and think about how attempting to convince a patient, who may have rigid and distorted thinking regarding taking any medication while breastfeeding, will likely not go far. Instead, you decide to examine the risk-assessment that you are making with her and understand her underlying thoughts and feelings behind taking escitalopram while breastfeeding using cognitive restructuring techniques. As Ms. P explicitly stated, you are aware that there is often a tension for mothers between wanting relief of their symptoms and not wanting to harm the infant, and that sometimes this is reinforced by stigma and misinformation of clinicians and patients. This tension is also likely exacerbated by Ms. P's symptoms, including her feelings of guilt that are a result of her depression as well as her anxiety, which may be amplifying the "threat" of medication. You discuss with Ms. P how her symptoms may be leading to a distorted view of the harms of medications while breastfeeding, and you ask for permission to describe some of the newer data regarding SSRIs while breastfeeding as a way to challenge these cognitive distortions as well as any misinformation she may have received from other sources. Ms. P says, "oh yeah, I remember that skill of challenging cognitive distortions from my therapist, that's helped me before," and agrees. You begin by framing the discussion as a decision that has a potential impact whether she chooses to treat or not treat her depression. Postpartum depression can potentially impact social, emotional, and cognitive development in an infant as well as result in impaired bonding between an infant and caregiver. There are also associated risks of depression for the mother including impaired functioning, suicide, or infanticide [12]. You take a moment and reflect to yourself that disclosing these risks of untreated or undertreated illness as Ms. P had in the third trimester may worsen her already exacerbated guilty feelings. Therefore, you try to make an effort to maintain a hopeful and forward-looking tone while at the same time being careful to not withhold information Ms. P needs to make her decision. To create a more positive framing, you also tell Ms. P that the way that you interpret this data is that caring appropriately for her own medical and psychiatric needs is an important part of caring effectively for her baby, and that whether she chooses to go back on an antidepressant or not, figuring out how to help her feel better is the most important part of her care. Regarding the risk of SSRIs, although there is limited long-term neurodevelopment data, overall SSRIs pass through the breast milk in low levels and have not been shown to have adverse effects in infants [4]. You discuss with Ms. P both sides of these risks, and given her trial of non-pharmacological interventions, the severity of her depression, the impact on bonding, and her new passive suicidal thoughts, you give your recommendation that the benefits of restarting escitalopram outweigh its risks at this point in time. She sighs, and asks you, "maybe if I just got a good night's sleep

I'd feel better? I heard that it's really common to have Postpartum Blues in your first two weeks…maybe that's all this is." You reply "that's a great question, and sometimes distinguishing between the two can be hard. For you, even though you are still within two weeks of delivery, the fact that you had symptoms during your third trimester, as well as the severity of your symptoms as indicated on the scale we did together, tells me this is a diagnosis of depression and not just blues" [12]. She nods and says, "that makes sense, what a relief really, I'm really happy to hear that there's so much information about this stuff…I guess I was seeing the medication as much more harmful than it is. All this information does make me feel better about restarting it." You provide the patient with information to access LactMed [4] so she can look up information on her own about different medications while breastfeeding, and help facilitate scheduling a follow-up appointment with her former outpatient psychiatrist.

You tell the OB/GYN resident your recommendation to restart her escitalopram prior to her being discharged and that she will follow up with her outpatient psychiatrist. The next day you follow up with Ms. P to make sure she tolerated the medication. When you get there she appears tearful and tells you she didn't end up starting the medication because the lactation consultant told her that it "really wasn't safe to take medications while breastfeeding" and she should try to "hold off" if she can. You tell Ms. P it sounds like hearing that touched on her own internal fears and anxieties, and that if it was okay with her you'd like to have a quick discussion with the lactation consultant to understand her concerns. You approach the lactation consultant and introduce yourself, and ask her about how things went with Ms. P. The lactation consultant says she went ahead and "counseled her that she really should try to see if she can get through this without medication since it's common to feel anxious and overwhelmed in the beginning – especially if it's your first child." The lactation consultant also adds that if she did need to start taking a medication, she read somewhere that sertraline was the "safest" and "best" SSRI to use while breastfeeding. Although your immediate impulse is to defend your and Ms. P's decision, one that required her to grapple with her own sense of shame, anxiety, and guilt, you think to yourself how the lactation consultant is giving recommendations that she believes are best for Ms. P and her infant and potentially based on her own more narrow focus on breastfeeding and the infant. You think about how her recommendations may stem from a duty she feels to "protect" the baby from perceived sources of harm, but are also aware of how this type of response contributes to the difficulties of mothers seeking out mental health care. You acknowledge the lactation consultant's point of view and validate her concerns while also providing her the same risk discussion and psychoeducation you provided to Ms. P. You also decide to quickly address the common myth the lactation consultant expressed that sertraline is the first-line and "safest" antidepressant to use for a woman who is breastfeeding, telling the lactation consultant that the "best" treatment, including medication, is the treatment that is most likely to reduce the patient's symptoms effectively. This takes into account many variables including the patient's prior treatment history, severity of symptoms, and relative safety risks of different medications and interventions. Reframing the medication safety discussion from the binary of "safe" or "not safe" to a process of weighing the relative risks of each peripartum exposure—both medication and maternal illness—can give the lactation consultant a more nuanced understanding of the decision Ms. P is making.

Being aware of the primary medical team and other ancillary staff's reactions to a mother taking psychiatric medication while breastfeeding or pregnant is important in implementation of your treatment recommendations. The psychiatric consultant can help anticipate delays in treatment or stigmatizing interactions with the patient that could lead to early and unnecessary cessation of breastfeeding, or to undertreatment of psychiatric symptoms. Stigma can be counteracted with psychoeducation that includes validation of any concerns in conjunction with highlighting the risks associated with untreated psychiatric illness. Other more subtle behaviors that may occur in the hospital and highlight the stigma of new mothers with psychiatric disorders include refusing to store expressed breastmilk from a mother taking psychiatric medications, or delays in getting a nursing mother access to a pump. Understanding the motivation behind these actions can help the psychiatric consultant preserve their patient's choices in treatment.

Appendix: Summary Table

	Problems	Strategies
• Patient symptoms and behaviors	• Waxing/waning symptoms and cognitive deficits associated with postpartum psychosis • Rapid onset of mood symptoms postpartum • Intrusive thoughts to harm baby or self or delusions involving new infant • Patient appears detached from baby • Guardedness misinterpreted as paranoia	• Offer specific psychoeducation regarding phenomenology of postpartum psychosis including delirium-like presentation such as cognitive effects and waxing/waning course of symptoms • Use validated scales for pregnancy and postpartum such as the Edinburgh Postnatal Depression Scale (EPDS) • Conduct safety assessment taking into account specific risks to infant including from psychosis • Ask patient directly about bonding and thoughts and feelings about infant; observe how the patient interacts with their infant • Understand patient's background including any history of trauma or discrimination to put patient's symptoms into context
• Provider-patient dynamics	• Provider has wish for mother to be healthy and to prevent mother-infant separation, leading to provider believing patient has improved or minimizing symptoms • Providers/staff may overly identify with baby and have wish to "protect" baby from mother	• Provide clear psychoeducation regarding the waxing/waning symptoms of postpartum psychosis • Advise team to provide pharmacologic interventions that weigh the risk of the psychiatric medication exposure during pregnancy or while breastfeeding with the risk of psychiatric illness itself to the mother and infant • Address staff member's assumptions regarding safety of medication in pregnancy by providing psychoeducation and online resources • Address desire of team to "protect" baby from mother by verbalizing the mother's autonomy in decision-making and providing materials counteracting belief that pharmacologic medication in pregnancy and while breastfeeding is harmful

• Inter-provider and provider-family dynamics	• Traumatized family member is fearful of medical doctors and does not want their family member to be psychiatrically hospitalized • Suspicion of mental health professionals by family that child will be taken away if a patient is given a psychiatric diagnosis or is seen by a mental health professional	• Engage family member in decision-making process and review symptoms that have led to decision to provide psychiatric treatment • Provide information regarding visiting hours, estimated lengths of admission, and how the doctors will be monitoring symptoms; involve any trusted members of the family's community including religious figures or community leaders • Educate family as to circumstances that would lead to the involvement of child protective services and what their role is • Validate and support distress over new diagnosis and impact of separation of infant and mother
• Patient-provider barriers	• Provider is uncomfortable providing diagnosis of postpartum psychosis due to implications on future pregnancies	• Provide standard of care to all patients, which should include providing a provisional diagnosis, treatment recommendations, and prognosis
• Hospital system barriers	• Patient would like to breastfeed or pump while on the inpatient psychiatric unit • Pharmacy may block prescribing medications to a pregnant woman based on outdated FDA labeling	• Familiarize yourself with the psychiatric inpatient unit's ability to provide contact with infant as well as pumping to provide patient with accurate information • Address any delays in nursing staff providing pump or ability to express stored milk for patient as a priority in patient care • Consider psychoeducation for inpatient pharmacy staff

References

1. Bergink V, Rasgon N, Wisner KL. Postpartum psychosis: madness, mania, and melancholia in motherhood. Am J Psychiatry. 2016;173(12):1179–88. https://doi.org/10.1176/appi.ajp.2016.16040454.
2. Bowlby J. The making and breaking of affectional bonds. Br J Psychiatry. 1977;130(3):201–10.
3. Hermann A, Gorun A, Benudis A. Lithium use and non-use for pregnant and postpartum women with bipolar disorder. Curr Psychiatry Rep. 2019;21(11):114. https://doi.org/10.1007/s11920-019-1103-3.
4. Drugs and Lactation Database (LactMed). 2019. https://toxnet.nlm.nih.gov/newtoxnet/lactmed.htm.
5. Viguera AC, Nonacs R, Cohen LS, Tondo L, Murray A, Baldessarini RJ. Risk of recurrence of bipolar disorder in pregnant and nonpregnant women after discontinuing lithium maintenance. Am J Psychiatry. 2000;157(2):179–84. https://doi.org/10.1176/appi.ajp.157.2.179.
6. Viguera AC, Whitfield T, Baldessarini RJ, Newport DJ, Stowe Z, Reminick A. Risk of recurrence in women with bipolar disorder during pregnancy: prospective study of mood stabilizer discontinuation. Am J Psychiatry. 2007;164(12):1817–24; quiz 923. https://doi.org/10.1176/appi.ajp.2007.06101639.
7. Bergink V, Armangue T, Titulaer MJ, Markx S, Dalmau J, Kushner SA. Autoimmune encephalitis in postpartum psychosis. Am J Psychiatry. 2015;172(9):901–8. https://doi.org/10.1176/appi.ajp.2015.14101332.
8. Postpartum Support International—PSI. 2020. https://www.postpartum.net/.
9. Wisner KL, Peindl KS, Gigliotti T, Hanusa BH. Obsessions and compulsions in women with postpartum depression. J Clin Psychiatry. 1999;60(3):176–80. https://doi.org/10.4088/jcp.v60n0305.
10. Abramowitz JS, Schwartz SA, Moore KM, Luenzmann KR. Obsessive-compulsive symptoms in pregnancy and the puerperium. J Anxiety Disord. 2003;17(4):461–78.
11. Mccabe-Beane JE, Segre LS, Perkhounkova Y, Stuart S, O'Hara MW. The identification of severity ranges for the Edinburgh Postnatal Depression Scale. J Reprod Infant Psychol. 2016;34(3):293–303. https://doi.org/10.1080/02646838.2016.1141346.
12. Stewart DE, Vigod S. Postpartum depression. N Engl J Med. 2016;375(22):2177–86. https://doi.org/10.1056/nejmcp1607649.

Further Reading

Bergink V, Burgerhout KM, Koorengevel KM, Kamperman AM, Hoogendijk WJ, Lambregtse-van den Berg MP. Treatment of psychosis and mania in the postpartum period. Am J Psychiatry. 2015;172(2):115–23. https://doi.org/10.1176/appi.ajp.2014.13121652.

7 Mood Disorders Secondary to a Medical Condition

Ariella R. Dagi and Jessica Daniels

Your pager reads: "The patient isn't sleeping — can we give him something?"

This page appears to be a simple request, but it does not lend itself to a straightforward answer. Initial questions to ask the consultant may attempt to establish an etiology for insomnia. For example, what are the patient's sleeping patterns? Is this a new, recurrent, or chronic problem? Was there a home medication or supplement that has been discontinued? What other symptoms have accompanied the poor sleep? Does the patient have any comorbid conditions that may be impacting quality or pattern of sleep, such as untreated sleep apnea, an exacerbation of congestive heart failure, or polyuria leading to increased nighttime awakenings to urinate? Other questions may address what has already occurred in the hospital. For example, primary medical teams are typically comfortable using a variety of medications for sleep. Has any medication already been trialed, and if not, is there a reason they are hesitant or unable to try their usual options? Have

A. R. Dagi
Department of Psychiatry, NewYork-Presbyterian Hospital/Weill Cornell Medicine, New York, NY, USA

J. Daniels (✉)
Adult Outpatient Behavioral Health, Baystate Medical Center, Springfield, MA, USA
e-mail: jessica.daniels@baystatehealth.org

A. Gorun et al. (eds.), *The Psychiatric Consult*,
https://doi.org/10.1007/978-3-031-26837-3_7

there been any interventions such as stat procedures at night or medications with the side effect of alertness that may have shifted sleep? It is also worth considering how the issue came to be a consult. Many patients experience at least partial insomnia in the hospital due to the noises, lights, blood draws, and vital signs checks, yet few cases of insomnia lead to psychiatric evaluation. While not specifically asked, the consult may also include questions about whether insomnia is related to a psychiatric condition, or how the insomnia may be affecting the patient's participation in or ability to receive care; the consult request may also convey the presence of a worried patient or family member who is advocating for additional resources or feels dissatisfied with care.

Clinical Scenario

You briefly look through the chart before answering the page, discovering that the patient, Mr. A, was diagnosed with prostate cancer a few months ago and, 4 days ago, presented with daily morning headaches concerning for central nervous system metastases. You take a peek at the vital signs, which have remained within normal range. You peruse the list of medications administered and see that he has been given a couple of doses of diphenhydramine and one dose of zolpidem. There are no other anxiolytics or sedatives on the list.

You call back the medical resident. She states that the team wants a recommendation on what to give him to sleep given that their usual go-tos have not worked. When you ask more about the clinical picture, she says that although definitive staging is not yet complete, Mr. A's prognosis is very poor. The team is awaiting imaging results prior to arranging a "goals of care" conversation with the patient and family. The resident says she feels "very bad" for the patient and has tried to accommodate his requests knowing that his time is limited, but it has become increasingly difficult to manage his demands. She mentions that when she conducted his initial admission, Mr. A was calm and pleasant, but in the last couple of days, she has witnessed him yelling at staff and even snapping at the attending. You hear a call in the background and she abruptly apologizes, stating she has to present another patient on rounds and concludes with, "I think he really just needs to sleep. That would probably help his mood."

Scenario 1: Steroid-Induced Hypomania

You go back to the chart after your conversation with the resident. You discover that since the first night of the admission the patient was newly placed on 16 mg of dexamethasone daily, considered a high dose of steroids, in addition to his pre-existing chemotherapy regimen [1, 2]. You see that he has been sent down to radiology twice, both in the very early hours of the morning, and that one of the studies had to be aborted due to the patient's inability to sit still enough to capture a high-quality image. Nursing notes indicate the patient has been pacing over the last couple of nights. An "event note" from overnight states that Mr. A started yelling at a nurse for not bringing him ice quickly enough, though he ultimately calmed down after speaking with the on-call resident. Daily follow-up notes indicate the patient has raised his voice at least twice during rounds. You begin to develop a picture of the dynamic at play among Mr. A, the nursing staff, and the primary team. As Mr. A has slept little and become irritable and restless, the nursing staff feel worn down by his non-urgent demands, and the primary team feels overwhelmed by what seem to be distractions from his oncologic care as well as saddened by his prognosis.

With this dynamic in mind, you go to see Mr. A. On the way over, you stop by the nursing station to see if you can catch any of the overnight staff before they head home. You run into the charge nurse who gives a big sigh when you mention Mr. A's name. She says that while just a few nights ago he was being joked about as the "prince charming" of the ward for making puns and chatting up the nurses' aides, Mr. A has since been barely sleeping, pacing the halls, and yelling at staff. She says, "I don't know what went wrong but my night crew have many patients to care for and need to be able to get their work done. That man needs to sleep!" You thank her for her time and input. You leave the nursing station, and she chimes in a "good luck" as you walk toward the patient's room.

Upon entering Mr. A's room, you notice papers messily stacked atop all available surfaces. There are bits of food and articles of clothing strewn about. He looks disheveled and has big bags under his eyes but is busily chatting with his roommate, who is facing away from him and appears to be trying to sleep. You start to introduce yourself but before you can finish stating why you have come, he launches into a complaint about the staff and asks if you can have his room changed. You find yourself wondering if you might be able to arrange this and realize he has elicited from you a wish to assist him. In any case, he does not let you get a word in, and a rush of annoyance hits you. You realize you have identified your counter transference: the desire to help accompanied by frustration that he will not let you. This counter transference seems to fit with the experience of the primary team, as well.

You finally manage to state your role and ask him about his sleep. He responds that he has not been able to get any sleep recently but then says he actually feels fine without it, despite his family's concern. You clarify that he has no psychiatric history and he has never had insomnia. He says he feels quite good and believes the cancer treatment must be going in the right direction based on the amount of energy he has. He then asks you to move aside, grabs a stack of papers and pen from his bedside table, and says he must get back to his work. As a wave of frustration returns, you are more convinced that the primary team has experienced a similar counter-transference.

You go back to the call room to find the medicine resident and convey your concern that Mr. A may be hypomanic, likely due to the high-dose steroids, which fits with the timeline of the presenting complaints (see Table 7.1 on risk factors for the development of steroid-induced neuropsychiatric symptoms) [3, 4]. You tell the resident you would like to discuss medication options with your attending but in the meantime would appreciate if he could discuss with his team the minimum dose and time frame of steroid treatment. You validate the team's frustration and provide supportive comments regarding the difficulty of balancing differing patient, family, and nursing staff expectations. You also mention the potential for feelings of helplessness given that the very treatment for the advancing cancer has brought on hypomanic symp-

Table 7.1 Risk factors for the development of steroid-induced neuropsychiatric symptoms

• **Risk factors**
Higher effective dose of corticosteroids is associated with the development of neuropsychiatric symptoms generally
Rapid titration of corticosteroids is associated specifically with hypomania or mania
Long course of corticosteroids is associated specifically with depression
• **Possible risk factors associated with the development of neuropsychiatric symptoms while on steroids (conflicting research or still undergoing study)**
Female sex
Hypoalbuminemia (marker of blood brain barrier disruption)
Age (older age may correlate with different symptoms than younger age)
• **Surprising pearls**
Pre-existing psychiatric history is *not* known to be an independent risk factor for the development of neuropsychiatric symptoms on corticosteroids, except for those with a history of PTSD, who were found to be at higher risk for the development of depression
Prior exposure to corticosteroids without experiencing side effects does *not* appear to be *protective* against the development of neuropsychiatric side effects with subsequent exposures

References: Ismail et al. [3] and Kenna et al. [4]

toms, which, in turn, make Mr. A clinically more difficult to manage. You also provide some psychoeducation on the common features of hypomania and treatment strategies for the inpatient setting, including behavioral strategies such as clear limit and expectation setting as well as the utility of short-term benzodiazepines to manage sleep (see Table 7.2 on management strategies for mania or hypomania on non-psychiatric units).

By providing the team with this information, you are giving them the answer to their original question about sleep as well as offering larger framework to understand and treat the patient holistically. Once you come back to them after discussing the case with your attending, you attend a brief meeting run by the team with Mr. A and his family to explain why he has been different from usual. The team is able to provide a treatment plan based on

Table 7.2 Management strategies for steroid-induced hypomania or mania

Common symptoms	Behavioral strategies	Medications
• Insomnia	• Establish bedtime schedule and employ sleep hygiene techniques • Minimize nighttime interruptions (e.g., decrease vitals checks, cluster necessary interactions)	• Dose corticosteroids in the morning • If medically appropriate, consider decrease in dose or duration of steroid course • Offer benzodiazepine, noting potential interactions with other medications
• Talking rapidly and loudly, frequent interruptions to staff	• Set limits around acceptable behavior clearly and consistently • Set reasonable expectations and create explicit plan for communication with team members	• Decrease or discontinue corticosteroid if risks of behaviors outweigh benefits of steroid treatment • Introduce a mood stabilizer such as lithium or divalproex, both of which can be given in a loading dose to achieve therapeutic level quickly; note necessary screening labs required to ensure safety and the potential for interactions with other medications • Introduce an antipsychotic; if severe behavioral disturbance is present, consider haloperidol or olanzapine, which can be administered via intramuscular injection; if insomnia is present, consider olanzapine or quetiapine dosed at nighttime
• Disorganized thought process when speaking to team members	• Encourage patient to invite a support person to be present for major conversations • Encourage the patient to write down concerns on one page • Team should use visual and written communication to facilitate communication	
• Impulsive or potentially dangerous behavior, e.g., pulling lines, running down hallways, entering others' rooms, attempting elopement	• Set and enforce clear expectations regarding behavior • Remove all potential safety hazards such as sharps containers from the room • Consider placement on 1:1 with staff	
• Poor reality testing; poor assessment of risks due to grandiosity	• Encourage patient to invite a friend or family member to be present for major conversation • Evaluate capacity for specific decisions as needed	

your recommendations, which, in turn, makes Mr. A and his family feel more comfortable that their concerns are being addressed and more confident in the medical team's care.

As you complete the note for the case that day, you think back on the development of the consultation. It began with the initial question about sleep that left open questions about underlying diagnosis. A conversation with the medicine resident revealed feelings of sadness over Mr. A's prognosis competing with frustration with his irritability and demands. The charge nurse's description of the patient's transformation from charming to aggravating helped contextualize the case. Finally, your own experience with the patient, in which you identified your hurt and impatience in response to the patient's help-seeking help-rejecting behavior and hyper-verbal speech.

Thinking back on the day, you realize that each of these steps provided crucial information to track the clinical change and discover the role of the high-dose steroids. You also recognize that your own counter transferential reactions to Mr. A, both positive and negative, helped you relate to the team's and nurses' experiences and enabled you to formulate a response to them that both supported their empathy and gave them a sense of agency in a situation that was beginning to feel dire. This strengthened the team's therapeutic alliance with Mr. A and his family, paving the way for the mutual trust required for successful cancer treatment as well.

Scenario 2: Cancer Pain-Induced Insomnia

You return to the chart after your conversation with the resident. You notice that the patient is written for a pain regimen of pro re nata (PRN) oxycodone 5 mg/acetaminophen 325 mg q12hours, which he has been getting regularly. You see that he was initially given two doses of morphine IV in the ED, listed as given for severe headache, but once he was transferred to the inpatient unit, he only received oral analgesia as above. You see a few subjective and objective pain scales filled out in the nursing flow sheets section, which indicate that while the patient described his pain as an

8 or 9, the nurses often rated objective pain at a 4 or 5. You are curious about the discrepancy in scores. Armed with this new data, you make your way to the patient's unit.

Once on the floor, you stop at the primary team's call room to check in with the resident about the team's perception of the patient's pain. You catch the resident furiously typing a note while simultaneously peering at and shooting off responses to pages and ask if you can briefly chat. She says "sure, but I only have a sec," so you quickly say you noticed some pain scales in the chart that say he has a score of 8, hoping that this might be a neutral enough opening to allow the resident to feel comfortable expressing her perspective candidly. Indeed, she scrunches her nose and says, "Ugh, I'm not really sure what to do. Mr. A often asks for more pain meds but he never actually looks like he is uncomfortable, and whenever I go back and check on him he seems fine and doesn't bring it up again until the next day. I mean he has cancer so I am fine giving him pain meds but it just doesn't seem like he actually needs them. My attending fears he might be drug seeking." You nod and say, "it seems like a difficult situation," and tell her you'll swing back around after seeing Mr. A.

As you enter his room you observe Mr. A in bed appearing to read, but on closer look you see he is fidgeting and lying in an awkward position. You introduce yourself and say the team has asked you to come by to help with his difficulty sleeping. Mr. A lets out a short laugh and says, "Yeah, I'm sure that's what *they* are worried about." Sensing some discrepancy in the team's and patient's goals, you pull your seat a little closer and ask Mr. A how he feels his care has been going overall. He says that it was terrifying to come into the hospital, which he had to be convinced to do by his family. Initially, though the ED was overwhelmingly busy, they were able to make his horrible headaches better, but in the last few days, it seems like the doctors don't care about his head and just want to keep pricking and poking him. He says he never wanted to be the kind of person to ask for pain medications – he has a few friends from childhood who ended up addicted to drugs and has always stayed away from all "vices," including refusing pain medications after knee and hip surgeries – but now that he feels like his head is exploding, no one seems to offer him anything to help. He wonders if he should have just stuck it out at home, where at least he would have been in his own bed. Here, he can't seem to sleep at all. Initially he tried to make friends with the nurses, but now he is so tired he can't help but get irritable at them, since they don't even seem to want to give him the pain medications he is ordered to have. He says that the medications help for only 4–5 h, so he spends the next 6–7 h in increasing pain, with the early morning hours being the worst. He sheepishly tells you he yelled at a young nurse last night and feels terrible about it.

You ask him some basic screening questions regarding his psychiatric history, to which he quickly answers "no" across the board. He also denies substance use and any prior history of insomnia. Mr. A says recently he has barely slept not only because of the headaches but also because of his worry that his pain will worsen but not be taken seriously. While speaking with him, you are aware of feeling bad for him and somewhat guilty that his pain is not being adequately managed despite hospitalization. Then, you become aware of some anger and you find yourself wondering if he is being honest with you about the substance use history as you realize how easily he answered "no" to all of your screening questions. You make a mental note that these seem to be the polarities that the resident expressed feeling, and feel more at ease as you find you can both interview the patient and observe the patterns of interaction as if from above. As you wrap up your interview, you pause to ask permission to speak with his family, which he provides, thinking that it would be useful to discuss any history of addiction. You tell Mr. A that you appreciate his openness and will return with the attending to speak further.

On the way out of his room, you quickly look up oxycodone/acetaminophen on UpToDate to remind yourself of the half-life. As you suspected, the half-life is only 3.5 h [5]. Although the extended release (ER) formulation is commonly dosed every 12 h, he is written for the immediate release (IR) formulation, which is often given every 4–6 h. You also log onto a computer at the nursing station to check Mr. A on the state prescription monitoring program and confirm that no controlled substances have been prescribed in your state or any of the neighboring states. You call your attending to update her, and she tells you she is just down the hall. You review the case and see Mr. A together. The attending agrees that Mr. A's insomnia appears to be from undertreated pain. She tells you about the concept of "pseudoaddiction" [6, 7], a clinical scenario in which the undertreatment of pain, often in the setting of concern for a substance use disorder, leads a patient to escalate pain-associated behaviors and medication requests in order to ensure appropriate analgesia, leading to a breakdown in trust between the treaters and the patient [6]. You acknowledge the existence of some controversy and develop some safe methods for ameliorating this iatrogenic dynamic, including increasing the availability of pain medications with clear parameters for dispensing them for mild, moderate, and severe pain and the capacity to make changes as needed [7]. As you discuss this, you realize you will have to bring up this topic to the team with caution and sensitivity, having yourself felt the suspicion and uncertainty that they expressed.

You return to the call room and find the medicine resident, who is now sitting with the whole team. You tell them you have spoken with Mr. A and indeed see that sleep has been a major issue, supporting their initial reason for the consult. You also convey your understanding that his poor sleep has manifested in irritability and demands at all hours of the night, placing a strain on the nursing staff and the night float residents. You briefly review that insomnia can be due to a myriad of issues and that typically treatments targeted at the etiology are most effective. You note that they made reasonable and commonly effective choices of diphenhydramine and zolpidem and that you agree a different approach is needed. With this lead in, you introduce the idea that perhaps pain may be playing a role. You state that you yourself were concerned about the potential for substance-seeking behaviors, validating their own concerns. After seeing Mr. A, reviewing the prescription monitoring program and the notes from this as well as prior admissions, you feel relatively confident that the patient is not regularly on pain medications and has consistently denied substance use issues. Furthermore, you think that if insomnia may be secondary to pain, other agents are unlikely to work and are more likely to lead to yet another night of frustration for all. You ask whether they are open to the idea of trialing a period of increased frequency of dosing of the medication they already have on board as well as adding a PRN medication for lower intensity pain, such that Mr. A would have an option for intervention at each level of pain. You suggest that even a couple of days of this approach, with the potential to involve psychiatry in a meeting or to enlist the help of the pain service, could help rebuild trust and actually make the patient, and the pain, easier to deal with. Although members of the team initially appear a little annoyed, they seem to warm to the idea of a trial of a different pain medication approach, especially when you say you will continue to follow Mr. A and can provide alternative strategies to address sleep if this does not work. You leave the call room feeling more hopeful.

You check in the next morning and learn that Mr. A slept at least 5 h and was much less irritable during morning rounds. The team feels comfortable with the adjusted medication regimen. They are already thinking about the next steps in the cancer care. You stop by Mr. A's room, too. He looks cheerful and he tells you he feels much better having slept overnight. Thinking back, you believe that the crux of the case was not the change in medication but rather in the shift that occurred through acknowledgement and support. The use of both the consultative and liaison roles was crucial to honestly assessing Mr. A's concerns and anticipating and validating the team's fears. These permitted the trial of changes that led to a full night of analgesia and sleep, stepping toward a restoration of therapeutic alliance.

Scenario 3: Cancer-Related Adjustment Disorder with Depressed/Anxious Mood

After getting the initial page, you look at the chart to see if you can find any other hints as to what might be going on. There are no notable medications, just the patient's outpatient chemotherapy regimen, which has been the same for the last week. There is no indication of any change in symptomatology other than acute headaches, which per the pain, flow sheets are well treated with just one dose of acetaminophen in the morning. The patient has been through a number of diagnostic tests, such as imaging and a lumbar puncture, some of which are still pending results but so far have been unremarkable.

You go see Mr. A in his room. When you arrive, you see that the lights are off and he is staring into space. He appears dysphoric and disheveled. You introduce yourself and your role, and he immediately says, "I'm not crazy. I just can't sleep." You ask him to describe what has been going on and for how long. You also ask him additional open-ended questions to see what else might be bothering him. He tells you that over the last week since he started having morning headaches, he has been convinced that his "borrowed time is up," that he must not have long to live. He thought he was given another chance at life with his cancer treatment, but now he imagines the worst as he awaits the test results. He couldn't sleep for a few nights leading up to the hospitalization, though when he first arrived at the unit, he was feeling more hopeful that there could be treatment options left for his cancer, so he was more upbeat and friendly. Now that a few days have passed and he has not heard any good news, he is terrified this could be the end. He feels down and irritable but is also embarrassed that his anger has gotten the better of him with his family and the staff. He timidly suggests that it is easier to bicker than to cry, which he worries would elicit pity, the idea of which he hates. He barely has an appetite. When he tries to sleep, his brain "just won't turn off," and he experiences intrusive images of financial and emotional difficulties his family will face when he is gone. He cannot seem to enjoy anything anymore, even the junky spy novels his son brought that he usually reads in one sitting. His kids are worried about his sleep more than anything else, it seems, and he expresses relief that they seem less aware of his fear. When you ask about suicidality, he says he still wants to live very much but simply does not believe that is likely to be a possibility. You conduct a mini-mental status exam, which he completes with ease. You thank him for his time and tell him you will speak with the team and get back to him.

You find your way to the resident call room to discuss the case. You find the intern and resident caring for Mr. A and share your impression that he may have an adjustment disorder with depressed mood, conveying that he is despondent over what he believes is likely the progression of his cancer. This is manifesting in insomnia, which appears to be the primary symptom he is expressing to the team and that the family is worried about, but you also noted irritability, dysphoria, hopelessness, anhedonia, and poor appetite on your evaluation. You discuss a few pharmacologic options that could address sleep and potentially perk up Mr. A's appetite and mood, such as mirtazapine, an atypical antidepressant thought to improve mood through blockade at adrenergic receptors but also with sedative properties due to a high affinity at histaminic [8]. You also make some suggestions regarding involvement of nutrition to obtain food preferences and enlist his family in behavioral activation. You convey that you are happy to provide psychoeducation along with the team to Mr. A and his family to help guide them through the changes they may see and provide support if there are any care decisions they consider. You also recommend that if Mr. A is interested, he may be a good candidate for Meaning-Centered Psychotherapy or Supportive-Expressive Therapy and then mention Family-Focused Grief Therapy as an additional option, for which you can provide referrals [9–11]. You say you may be able to start this process by providing daily 45-min psychotherapy sessions with Mr. A during the hospital course. You also recommend they consider his spiritual needs and enlist the help of chaplaincy.

You return to your shared office with the other psychiatry residents on the consult-liaison service. You find yourself thinking about Mr. A and his family, feeling a sadness for the situation they are in and identifying with them strongly. You consider the time you spent with the team and realize you may have offered so many different psychotherapeutic suggestions and options as a defense against your own feelings of helplessness in the face of a rapidly progressing cancer in a patient whom you found quite likable. You decide to discuss this with your attending in rounds later, realizing it is likely neither feasible nor your role as a rotator on an inpatient consult-liaison team to provide daily 45-min psychotherapy sessions. You hope to develop a greater awareness of this internal response in order to hone your clinical skills and to recognize in what clinical situations you may be most vulnerable to burnout due to offering services that do not match the context of treatment.

Appendix: Summary Table

	Problems	Strategies
• Patient symptoms and behaviors	• Affective: Irritability, lability • Cognitive: Poor memory, decreased attention span, risk for delirium • Behavioral: Agitation, refusal to participate or poor engagement in care	• Assist with diagnostic clarification and support the team in identifying and addressing underlying etiology of insomnia • Provide guidance in minimizing iatrogenic and environmental contributions to insomnia • Offer easy-to-follow management recommendations, including behavioral and environmental strategies to support sleep and prevent development of delirium • Consider pharmacologic interventions for managing insomnia based on etiology and help guide avoidance of polypharmacy that may increase the patient's risks of side effects or the development of delirium
• Provider-patient dynamics	• Provider may have feelings of frustration either that patient is complaining of something they do not perceive to be a major issue or that patient is intrusive or irritable as a result of insomnia. May mobilize defensive sense of anger and disengagement, feelings of being undervalued or poorly treated, or be projected onto patient as being aggressive • Patient may have irritability and be demanding or intrusive with staff, which contributes to staff frustration, sense of disempowerment, avoidance, over-medication, or use of polypharmacy. Additionally, patient may have concerns about being perceived as medication-seeking that may prevent them from having sough care at an earlier stage when the problem may have been more mild	• Attempt to establish a clear etiology to guide more directed and therefore effective treatment strategies • Re-engage them in medical workup and management as it pertains to or is affected by insomnia • Outline active interventions and appropriate boundaries to help the patient and re-empower the team • Validate and empathize with team frustrations and concerns while supporting their continued thoughtful care for the patient

• Inter-provider and provider-family dynamics	• Team may attribute insomnia to an underlying psychiatric disorder (e.g., bipolar disorder, primary insomnia), leading to sense of being de-skilled, a drive to off-load patient's issue, and potential risk of missing medical or iatrogenic contributors or causes of insomnia • Family distressed about insomnia, that treatments have been ineffective, or the perception that the primary team is underplaying the importance of insomnia	• Attempt to establish a clear etiology for insomnia and provide accompanying psychoeducation for the primary team and family. May remark explicitly if there are no primary psychiatric comorbidities or contributions to current presentation • Assist in guiding and expanding primary team's thinking about the etiology further workup of the insomnia to re-engage • Consider continuing to follow and consult on the patient after evaluation to collaborate and provide team with support • Educate family about insomnia and expectations regarding sleep in the hospital context as well as in use of behavioral strategies and judiciously using pharmacologic strategies to address sleep. Support family in their distress
• Patient-provider barriers	• Poor patient health literacy regarding their health status and workup may lead patient to misunderstandings regarding the approach being taken for insomnia	• Provide patients with poor health literacy with clear, simple, and concrete explanations, ideally in both written and verbal format. Identify and elicit support from family or next of kin • Assist primary team in identifying key areas for therapeutic alliance building and if there are crucial pieces information still needed; offer to obtain collateral from patient's psychiatric providers, if relevant
• Hospital system barriers	• Patient may need to share a room with others • Staffing may not be able to support clustering nighttime events for all patients • Limited time of primary providers with patients may be a hurdle in establishing rapport, conducting timely family meetings, or conveying psychoeducation in the ideal manner	• Advocate for appropriate allocation of single rooms and use of privacy curtains in shared rooms • Set aside time in the consultation for liaising with nursing staff and primary team • Offer to assist in psychoeducation of the patient or family

References

1. Ryken TC, McDermott M, Robinson PD, Ammirati M, Andrews DW, Asher AL, Burri SH, Cobbs CS, Gaspar LE, Kondziolka D, Linskey ME, Loeffler JS, Mehta MP, Mikkelsen T, Olson JJ, Paleologos NA, Patchell RA, Kalkanis SN. The role of steroids in the management of brain metastases: a systematic review and evidence-based clinical practice guideline. J Neurooncol. 2010;96(1):103–14.
2. Buttgereit F, Silva Da JAP, Boers M, Burmester GR, Cutolo M, Jacobs J, Kirwan J, Kohler L, Riel P, van Vischer T, Bijlsma JWJ. Standardised nomenclature for glucocorticoid dosages and glucocorticoid treatment regimens: current questions and tentative answers in rheumatology. Ann Rheum Dis. 2002;61:718–22.
3. Ismail MF, Lavelle C, Cassidy EM. Steroid-induced mental disorders in cancer patients: a systematic review. Future Oncol. 2017;13(29):2719–31.
4. HA Kenna & AW Poon, 2011, de los Angeles CP, Koran LM. Psychiatric complications of treatment with corticosteroids: review with case report, Psychiatry Clin Neurosci, 65, 6, 549–560.
5. Oxycodone and acetaminophen (paracetamol): Drug information. In: Post TW, editor. UpToDate [database on the internet]. Waltham, MA: UpToDate; 2014. Updated 17 Dec 2019. http://www.uptodate.com. Accessed 30 Jan 2020.
6. Weissman DE, Haddox JD. Opioid pseudoaddiction—an iatrogenic syndrome. Pain. 1989;36(3):363–6.
7. Greene MS, Chambers RA. Pseudoaddiction: fact or fiction? An investigation of the medical literature. Curr Addict Rep. 2015;2(4):310–7.
8. Hirsch M, Birnbaum RJ. Atypical antidepressants: pharmacology, administration, and side effects. In: Roy-Byrne PP, Solomon D, editors. UpToDate. Waltham, MA: UpToDate; 2020. Updated 31 May 2018. http://www.uptodate.com. Accessed 1 Apr 2020.
9. Breitbart WS, Poppito SR. Individual meaning-centered psychotherapy for patients with advanced cancer: a treatment manual, vol. 1. New York: Oxford University Press; 2014.
10. Masterson MP, Schuler TA, Kissane DW. Family focused grief therapy: a versatile intervention in palliative care and bereavement. Bereave Care. 2013;32(3):117–23.
11. Daniels J, Kissane DW. Psychosocial interventions for cancer patients. Curr Opin Oncol. 2008;20(4):367–71.

8 Somatic Symptom Disorder

Christian Umfrid and Anna Dickerman

The pager reads: "The workup is negative, are the patient's symptoms psychological?"

Consultations related to somatic symptoms are typically prompted by one of two broad concerns: that the patient's perception of—or psychological response to—somatic symptoms may be maladaptive or pathological, or that the medical signs and symptoms themselves are produced by a psychological process rather than "organic" medical pathology. In cases in which the primary team is seeking assistance with the patient's response to somatic symptoms, clarifying the question will involve identifying the nature and duration of the symptoms, with particular attention to the ways in which they are causing distress—are they interfering with patient care or disposition? In what ways are they affecting the functioning of the patient or medical team? Is the distress being experienced entirely by the patient, or also by those involved in the patient's care? Information on how the patient is interacting with the team will be useful to obtain, as patient distress may manifest behaviorally and interpersonally in

C. Umfrid (✉)
Weill Cornell Medicine, New York-Presbyterian Hospital, New York, NY, USA

A. Dickerman
Department of Psychiatry, New York-Presbyterian Hospital/Weill Cornell Medicine, New York, NY, USA

A. Gorun et al. (eds.), *The Psychiatric Consult*,
https://doi.org/10.1007/978-3-031-26837-3_8

ways that are challenging for the team to manage while delivering care.

When there is suspicion that medically unexplained symptoms are functional in nature, the consult usually takes the form of a request for assistance with diagnostic confirmation or to evaluate for comorbid psychiatric conditions which may be impacting the patient's presentation or course of treatment. What may be prompting the request, however, may be more complex concerns or wishes—perhaps related to patient disposition, the providers' feelings of defeat, or an understandable hope for a psychiatric solution to a complex and potentially disabling cluster of symptoms. Common themes that may emerge upon initial interaction with the team include negative countertransference toward the patient, anxiety and uncertainty in the delivery of a psychiatric diagnosis, as well as hopelessness and frustration about the lack of identified medical diagnoses and being tasked to treat symptoms without a clear somatic etiology.

Clinical Scenario

You return the primary team's page and learn that the patient, Ms. A, is a previously healthy 26-year-old woman with a history of epilepsy in childhood, who presented to the emergency department with her husband 3 days ago, concerned that she was experiencing a recurrence of seizures. Ms. A reported multiple spontaneous episodes of staring over the course of 2 weeks, frequently preceded by a sense of being "confused and shaky" and vague changes in her vision. Each episode was accompanied by an apparent altered level of consciousness and followed by inter-episode anxiety and concentration difficulties.

Ms. A experienced one of these events prior to her presenting to the hospital, and her husband expressed concern that her symptoms were progressively worsening. Prior to her admission to the hospital, Ms. A had spontaneously fallen to the ground while at home and had a prolonged period in which she was unresponsive to her husband's voice, accompanied by abnormal movement of her extremities and urinary incontinence. There was no evidence of a head strike, tongue biting, or other injury sustained during the episode. By the time Ms. A had arrived at the emergency department, she was asymptomatic, and her subsequent medical workup—including labs, EKG, and non-contrast head CT—was "largely unremarkable" per the primary team. Her neurologic exam demonstrated no focal deficits.

The medical resident explains that Ms. A has been anxious and demanding since admission and has become distressed each time the team has outlined a plan to discharge her with outpatient follow-up. The resident notes that Ms. A's workup has been negative, yet she is refusing discharge and expressing a desperate worry that the team is "missing something." The primary team feels that Ms. A is struggling with "depression and anxiety" and wonders if her medical symptoms are psychological in nature or related to underlying psychopathology, better suited to treatment on an inpatient psychiatric unit.

Scenario 1: Somatic Symptom Disorder

Review of Ms. A's charted history reveals that she had taken antiepileptic drugs throughout early childhood for seizures related to a cerebral arteriovenous malformation (AVM). Her neurologist stopped these medications in adolescence following AVM resection and a sustained seizure-free period, and Ms. A had not experienced recurrence of seizures in the interim. Her workup during this hospitalization has been unremarkable for toxic, metabolic, or infectious etiologies of syncope, seizures, and her changes in mental status; her head imaging was normal, her history and urine drug screen did not indicate recent substance use, and she is not taking any medications that can affect seizure threshold. At the time of consultation, Ms. A has been on telemetry to rule-out cardiogenic syncope, and is undergoing video electroencephalogram (EEG), thus far without epileptiform activity.

Documentation of outpatient care is available in Ms. A's chart, and you note that she has had numerous visits to her neurologist and primary care physician over the past year, a marked increase in medical care-seeking relative to years prior. You briefly review the notes for recent changes that may provide clues to her current presentation or seizure recurrence—Ms. A is noted to be generally healthy, with no documented seizures, neurologic injuries or deficits, and no changes in her outpatient medication regimen. What does stand out in an otherwise unremarkable outpatient chart is that each visit was initiated by the patient, and for a specific concern—headaches, dizziness and lightheadedness, unusual visual phenomena, and paresthesias. These visits prompted diligent, negative, and often redundant medical and neurologic testing. This type of exhaustive and repetitious diagnostic approach commonly occurs when patients present with a high burden of somatic symptoms and carries its own risk for iatrogenic harm and patient distress. Each visit in Ms. A's chart concluded with notation that "reassurance was provided" and multiple medications have been trialed for symptom management. You see that anxiety was added to Ms. A's problem list, without further elaboration or treatment.

You call the primary resident and he asks about treating Ms. A's anxiety. You probe further to get a sense for what behavior the medical team is interpreting as anxiety. The resident reports that Ms. A has been refusing to engage in discharge planning and becomes acutely anxious when the team mentions discontinuing the workup and discharging her home. He tells you that Ms. A has been demanding to speak to him frequently regarding a variety of vague symptoms or to review the results of her medical evaluation, including those already explained to her in great detail. Ms. A has been repeatedly seeking reassurance from the medical team and nurses, and the resident tells you that such reassurance "doesn't help, she's convinced that there is something wrong," despite her exam and workup being normal. The resident reports that Ms. A has been requesting a brain MRI, but that this is not indicated as she has had extensive outpatient imaging and medical testing in recent months. The team feels that Ms. A has become angry, dissatisfied with her care, and "just won't listen" with each attempt to explain the rationale for their treatment decisions. He acknowledges that the team cannot fully rule out the presence of seizures given her concerning history and the absence of ictal episodes captured while monitored on video EEG, but he believes that her symptoms are related to or heightened by her anxiety. Indeed, he candidly shares his fear that "she is going to lose it" as she approaches discharge. You ask if Ms. A has agreed to meet with psychiatry, and the resident reluctantly informs you that he did not discuss the consultation with her as the team has not yet rounded on her that day, noting "it's impossible to get out of the room once I go in."

You speculate that Ms. A's anxiety and her perceived needy, demanding behavior may be escalating as a result of a sense of invalidation, feeling that her symptoms are being dismissed prematurely. This perception may have been primed by earlier experiences with fatigued and exasperated care providers. While the team's approach has included hospitalization and a thorough medical workup, you suspect that her response reflects the disconnect between her overwhelming, preoccupied health anxiety and the team's more rational and restrained response to her symptoms. You hypothesize that Ms. A may also be experiencing feelings of desperation and abandonment as the team has begun to pull away and avoid her in the setting of excessive demands, as well as their lack of diagnostic answers and waning patience.

You express concern to the resident that Ms. A may feel further alienated by the introduction of psychiatry without prior education about the indications and benefits of the consultation, and emphasize the importance of a tactful explanation of how psychiatric assessment may fit into her treatment plan. You highlight the importance of this to ensure that the patient feels that she has a role in her treatment, that her concerns are not being prematurely pathologized, and to maintain critical trust and rapport with her. You offer the resident guidance in his approach to sharing his concerns with Ms. A, recommending that he maintain and express empathy for her *experience* of the symptoms and their resultant distress. You also suggest that he emphasize the reciprocal relationship between psychosocial stressors and somatic symptoms. Another helpful frame for psychiatric consultation in patients like Ms. A is to introduce the role of psychiatry as a complementary and collaborative way of helping the patient manage and cope with symptoms, *in addition to*—not *instead of*—continued medical management. This approach aims to unify the psychological and the somatic, highlighting their close relationship with the goal of communicating optimism for the improvement of her physical symptoms with multimodal treatment [1]. The resident agrees and pages you after discussing the recommendation for psychiatric consultation with Ms. A.

You approach Ms. A in her hospital room and introduce yourself. She appears nervous and irritably interrupts you to note that "everyone thinks it's all in my head, but I'm not 'crazy.'" You express that you understand her concern and reassure her that no one believes her symptoms can be "cured" psychiatrically. Rather, you state that your goal is to collaborate with her other providers in an effort to help her manage symptoms. Indeed, patients are more open to psychiatric consultation when it is a part of an ongoing medical treatment plan [1]. You also emphasize that patients struggling with a high burden of physical symptoms may have difficulty coping and often struggle with anxiety or mood symptoms, making initial efforts to connect her distress primarily to her medical concerns. This implicitly allows her permission to discuss emotional symptoms without fear of being dismissed as "crazy." Ms. A's initial guardedness seems to soften over the course of your evaluation, as you establish rapport by emphasizing the physical distress, asking about her symptoms with neutrality, expressing interest in her experience of each symptom and the meaning she assigns them. You are careful to not prematurely overemphasize a contribution from psychological factors but rather to highlight how stressors may exacerbate her somatic symptoms, with the goal of prompting her to reflect on their relationship [2].

You complete a psychiatric evaluation aimed at identifying comorbidities, given the high co-occurrence of somatic distress with depressive and anxiety disorders [1]. Ms. A describes anxiety related to a variety of physical symptoms—headache, blurred vision, dizziness, paresthesias, nausea, fatigue, and heart palpitations—which she worries must be due to an underlying, undiagnosed neurologic disorder. She spends several hours daily researching medical conditions online and engaging in checking behaviors, including examining herself for neurologic signs and asymmetry, and periodically repeating a Valsalva maneuver in an effort to reproduce her headache and vision symptoms. You are struck by the degree of anxiety, time dedicated, and functional impairment she has experienced around her illness concerns. Through careful evaluation of the nature and context of her symptoms, you identify near-daily panic attacks which occur when she researches and ruminates on catastrophic diagnostic possibilities. You educate Ms. A on the symptoms of panic—many of which she has been misattributing to medical and neurologic pathology. Her misattribution of somatic phenomena underscores the role of interoceptive and perceptive dysfunction in somatic symptom disorder, as well as an important potential treatment target [2].

Although Ms. A's medical workup is ongoing, the disproportionate distress she has experienced is sufficient to make a diagnosis of somatic symptom disorder. Importantly, the diagnosis of somatic symptom disorder does not require the *absence* of underlying medical pathology [3]; in a shift away from historical mind-body dualism, the diagnosis instead focuses on the identification of maladaptive behaviors and distress experienced by the patient, rather than the lack of identified organic pathology. You discuss treatment options with Ms. A and recommend referral for psychotherapy, along with consideration of pharmacologic management with a selective serotonin reuptake inhibitor. Evidence for the treatment of somatic symptom disorder has demonstrated modest effects for psychotherapy—specifically short-term psychodynamic psychotherapy and cognitive behavioral-based therapies—and serotonergic antidepressants in both physical and psychiatric symptom reduction [4–6]. Your treatment recommendations also include regularly scheduled appointments for medical follow-up and consolidation of her medical management with her primary care physician. Ms. A agrees but worries her doctors are no longer interested in treating her, noting "I've asked to speak to them *again and again*, and they're all avoiding me."

Ms. A's husband is present and provides his insight and key collateral information. Per his observations, Ms. A became markedly more anxious following the unexpected death of her mother 1 year ago, after suffering an ischemic stroke. Ms. A insatiably seeks reassurance from her husband and seems to become dysregulated, "inconsolable and panicked" when she feels his response is inadequate, dismissive, or when he expresses his own frustration. Their relationship has become increasingly strained as a result. Childhood illness and trauma, concurrent psychiatric or medical diagnoses, psychosocial stressors, losses, and maladaptive coping strategies may contribute to the pathogenesis and perpetuation of somatic symptom disorders [1, 2]. Further, childhood adversity and an anxious attachment style are associated with somatic symptoms and high health anxiety in adulthood [7]. Although you have limited developmental history from Ms. A, you consider how she interacts with her husband and care providers and can begin to hypothesize about her somatization and behavioral changes over the past year. You speculate about the presence of an anxious attachment style and underlying abandonment concerns, heightened dependency needs with the recent loss of a significant object of attachment, and early traumatic experiences with a serious medical illness, all factoring in the use of maladaptive means of expressing somatic distress and eliciting care from others. You keep these considerations in mind as you guide the primary team in their interactions with Ms. A.

You meet with the team and emphasize the need for consistent, reliable follow-up from both inpatient and outpatient treatment providers. This is critical for reducing provider avoidance, which can elicit feelings of being dismissed and abandoned, as well as minimizing the perception that care is dependent on the presence of physical symptoms [2]. You highlight the importance of providing continued empathic reassurance and acknowledging the patient's symptoms as a complex expression of distress [2]. You provide a referral for outpatient psychiatric care with the recommendation for psychotherapy and emphasize the importance of continued close collaboration between her psychiatrist and outpatient medical provider.

Scenario 2: Functional Neurological Symptom Disorder (Conversion Disorder)

You return the primary team's pager request, and the neurology resident describes the patient's hospital course, including her "needy and demanding behavior," apparent anxiety, and a critical diagnostic event that occurred shortly after initiating video EEG monitoring. After a complete medical workup—including unremarkable basic labs, urine toxicology screen, EKG and telemetry monitoring, non-contrast head CT, and a normal neurologic exam—the patient was started on video EEG monitoring. Shortly after the technician applied the EEG leads, Ms. A had an event that clinically resembled a seizure, as recorded on video and observed by a nurse who was attending to the patient. The resident informs you that Ms. A's EEG demonstrated a normal, alert background and alpha rhythm, with no epileptic focus or generalized epileptiform activity during or around this event—indicating that Ms. A had not had an epileptic seizure. The neurology team shared their diagnostic impression with Ms. A, noting that the results were reassuring as "the episodes are not real seizures, and are *only* psychological."

The primary team would like to discharge Ms. A with psychiatric follow-up; however, she has been objecting to the discharge, expressing concern that the team is dismissing her symptoms as "all in her head," insisting that they are incompetent and "must be missing something." You inquire about Ms. A's psychiatric and psychosocial history, and the neurology resident notes that she confirmed a history of "depression and anxiety" when prompted, but seemed defensive—brusquely asking "what does that have to do with anything?"—and the team felt uncomfortable and inhibited from inquiring further. The primary resident expresses that the team would like psychiatry's assistance with various aspects of Ms. A's diagnosis and management—diagnostic clarification and confirmation of psychogenic seizures, diagnosing a suspected anxiety disorder, and providing treatment and disposition recommendations. You frame the consultation as an assessment of suspected psychological factors contributing to the patient's neurologic symptoms, which must include an evaluation of major current and historical psychological stressors or trauma, along with a careful assessment for comorbid psychiatric and medical pathology.

The neurology team's leading diagnosis for Ms. A is psychogenic nonepileptic seizures (PNES), a specific subtype of functional neurological symptom disorder (FNSD) or conversion disorder [3]. Although this diagnosis is suspected by the primary team, your initial approach to the consultation involves maintaining an unbiased and broad differential diagnosis until further objectively informed; in the case of Ms. A, the differential includes physiologic nonepileptic symptoms (e.g., syncope, cataplexy and other signs of parasomnias, toxic or metabolic derangements), epileptic seizures or specific foci that may not be visible on EEG (e.g., simple partial seizures, frontal lobe seizures), malingering, factitious disorder, and panic disorder [8]. The diagnosis of FNSD is dependent on a clinical determination of symptoms being *incompatible* with neurologic pathophysiology, rather than a lack of neurologic diagnosis or identifiable organic etiology of the symptom; it is a diagnosis requiring inconsistency with neurologic dysfunction based on findings of the evaluation and history, rather than a diagnosis of exclusion . In suspected PNES, intra-episode EEG provides critical objective data to rule out most epileptic events; however, EEG findings must also be correlated with observations of seizure semiology along with history and a presentation that are collectively incompatible with epileptic seizures [9].

To understand the primary team's clinical reasoning, you ask the neurology resident about the findings on physical exam and the observations of Ms. A's ictal and postictal behavior. The resident tells you that Ms. A has had two seizure-like episodes since presenting to the hospital, one in the emergency department and one after initiating EEG monitoring, both observed by her husband and clinical staff. Ms. A's seizures were prolonged and persisted for close to 10 min, during which she was noted to be unresponsive to voice, her eyes were closed and she resisted attempts to open them during examination, and her motor activity fluctuated from flaccid to brief, dysrhythmic writhing of her extremities. During the first episode, Ms. A was noted to be rotating her head from one side to the other as the nurse examined her [10, 11]. Following resolution of each seizure episode, Ms. A rapidly returned to baseline without postictal confusion, amnesia, or lethargy and was able to recall staff attempting to get her attention, talking about her care among themselves, and administering medication. The team confirmed with Ms. A's husband that these observations were consistent with the episode that he had observed which prompted her initial presentation. The neurology resident adds that each of these clinical signs are reliable indicators of PNES, are uncommon in epileptic seizures, and further support their diagnostic impression [10, 11].

As you prepare to evaluate Ms. A, you consider the approach to a patient with functional neurological symptoms. Recalling Ms. A's defensive, angry response to the primary team's initial diagnostic discussion, you have an impression that the team's delivery and well-intentioned attempts at reassurance—focused on the organic pathology *not* present, without attending to the patient's functional symptoms and distress—and their early effort to link her symptoms to her psychiatric history may have been experienced by the patient as dismissive, accusatory, or even humiliating. You feel wary as the psychiatrist tasked to evaluate a patient who has not accepted the diagnosis of a functional disorder and who may see no role for your involvement, but steel yourself knowing that psychiatric evaluation is critical in this patient population. Psychotherapeutic interventions may reduce Ms. A's symptom burden, along with the risk for iatrogenic harm from unnecessary healthcare visits and medical interventions [12]. Importantly, the process of evaluating Ms. A—including a tactful discussion of her diagnosis and treatment recommendations—can also be therapeutic, helping to reduce symptom recurrence and future emergency room visits [13].

You approach Ms. A and she is in her hospital bed, still connected to EEG leads. Her husband is sitting at bedside, attending to her and appearing concerned. You introduce yourself and your role as the psychiatric consultant, and Ms. A appears immediately irritated, interrupting you to note "My doctors seem to think I'm making this up just because they can't figure out what's wrong with me...I don't need a shrink." You ask Ms. A about her understanding of the diagnosis, and why you were asked to meet with her—she explains that the primary team has not been able to identify the cause of her symptoms, so have concluded that "they're all in [her] head." As patients frequently find the diagnosis of PNES confusing, and a reaction to the diagnosis with anger and hostility predicts poorer outcomes [14], you see the consultation as an opportunity to provide Ms. A with psychoeducation and begin to shift her understanding and perception of the diagnosis. You respond to Ms. A's negative experience with empathy, noting that one of your goals is to help identify and address some of her concerns. You reframe the consultation by acknowledging that she is experiencing *real* and *distressing* symptoms—regardless of their etiology—and that you would like to better understand how the symptoms are affecting her, how she is coping with them, and any other stressors that she may be facing which could be impacting her health. In your evaluation, you make sure to initially spend time eliciting all of Ms. A's medical symptoms, including their onset and evolution, how they have affected her emotionally and functionally, as well as her thoughts, concerns, and conceptualization of them. This process is intended to facilitate gaining an understanding of the meaning of the physical symptoms to the patient, while building rapport prior to psychiatric inquiry [15].

Ms. A seems to appreciate your concern about her physical symptoms and becomes more comfortable talking to you as you demonstrate interest in her experience and acknowledge her distress. She shares with you that she has been concerned about having a serious medical illness for the past several months, as she has episodically felt "out of it and dizzy...aware of what's going on, but foggy, and like [her] body is out of [her] control." You recognize her description as consistent with dissociative symptoms, which are frequently associated with functional disorders and continue to assess for other unrecognized or misattributed psychiatric symptomatology [10]. Ms. A acknowledges a history of depressive and anxiety symptoms which have never been psychiatrically evaluated or treated and endorses several months of low mood, anhedonia, as well as a decline in sleep and appetite. She is quick to deny any antecedent stressors related to the occurrence of her convulsive episodes and is adamant that such factors are not relevant to her symptoms. However, patients with PNES often deny the existence of psychosocial stressors even when present and may minimize the impact of psychological distress on their neurological symptoms, instead viewing their symptoms as concretely somatic and beyond their control [16].

As you tactfully broaden the scope of the interview to assess other realms of the patient's life and functioning, she reveals that her relationship with her husband has been strained for many months and that they have recently begun to consider separating. You ask Ms. A about her husband's presence in the hospital, and she denies any negative feelings toward him, describing him as an important source of support. Ms. A casually remarks that, despite their conflicts, her husband has "remained by [her] side" and has been particularly worried about her well-being since her mother's sudden and unexpected death last year. You are struck by the disconnect between this revelation and Ms. A's earlier denial of stressors. You note Ms. A's use of isolation of affect—evident in the incongruity between the considerable recent conflict and losses she has endured and her apparent lack of distress and minimization of their impact—and wonder how this might be concretized as physical symptoms. You begin to conceptualize Ms. A's loss of important attachments—the death of her mother and threatened loss of her husband—as one potential precipitant of her nonepileptic seizures. Functional disorders, however, typically have a complex and multifactorial etiology and are often associated with concurrent or historical psychiatric and medical comorbidities (e.g., prior experiences of epileptic seizures), as well as major early-life trauma, including neglect, and sexual and physical abuse [9].

You ask the neurology resident to join you for additional discussion with Ms. A and her husband, understanding that provider biases, diagnostic uncertainty, and frustration can detrimentally impact how a functional disorder diagnosis is introduced to the patient. You explain to Ms. A that while her symptoms are real and understandably distressing to her, her medical evaluation has been reassuring, and there does not appear to be irreversible neurologic or medical pathology. You tell Ms. A explicitly that she is not having epileptic seizures and elaborate how the neurology team arrived at this conclusion, offering to review the EEG interpretation and medical workup together if additional clarity is needed; you reassure Ms. A that her symptoms can improve and that she can play an active role in the treatment. You conclude by acknowledging that stress can contribute to her physical symptoms and identify the significant dissociative and depressive symptoms that have also emerged in the setting of her multiple major stressors [15]. You recommend psychiatric follow-up, framing the treatment goals as supporting her recovery and helping her to cope with the symptoms she is experiencing as well as her other recent stressors. You convey optimism for treatment outcomes by explaining that there is evidence for cognitive behavioral therapy in reducing seizure recurrence, psychodynamic psychotherapy for reducing symptom burden and developing insight into the physical symptoms, and for antidepressant pharmacotherapy for comorbid depressive and anxiety disorders [17, 18]. Ms. A is amenable to considering psychiatric treatment and has begun to become more open to the idea that her physical symptoms, interpersonal conflict and losses, and psychological distress are interrelated. She accepts the referrals you provide her, is eager to leave the hospital, and is discharged later that day with close outpatient medical and psychiatric follow-up.

Scenario 3: Factitious Disorder

After receiving the consult request, you briefly review Ms. A's chart to familiarize yourself with her hospital course and medical workup. The pager question indicates that the team is concerned about psychological factors motivating Ms. A's presentation, so you are surprised to see that she has only recently been moved out of the medical intensive care unit; since admission, Ms. A has been undergoing blood glucose monitoring while on a continuous intravenous dextrose drip, after experiencing multiple episodes of severe hypoglycemia of unknown etiology.

Admission documentation reports that Ms. A's blood glucose was 22 mg/dL when she was found at home by paramedics—stuporous, diaphoretic, and postictal. Following administration of glucose in the field, Ms. A's blood glucose had increased to 82 mg/dL and she had become alert and was asymptomatic by the time she had arrived in the emergency department. You see from the medical team's notes—including "rapid response" documentation—that Ms. A has had two additional episodes of hypoglycemia while receiving IV fluids with dextrose; during the first she became agitated, confused, and tremulous, and during the second, she was found unresponsive, ultimately prompting her transfer to the intensive care unit. The patient has no other active medical problems and no documented psychiatric or substance use history. You search the chart for prior psychiatric consultation notes (there are none) and see that Ms. A has had three other emergency department visits over the past year—once for abdominal cellulitis and twice for milder symptoms of hypoglycemia. On her current presentation, she had requested to be admitted to the service of the attending physician who had previously treated her cellulitis, whom she spoke of in glowing and idealized terms. Documentation from multiple clinicians describe Ms. A as quite anxious, frequently demanding medication to treat disparate medical symptoms, asking for intravenous benzodiazepines for anxiety, and pushing for further diagnostic testing. She is noted to be hostile, belittling, and threatening toward nurses and the medicine resident when they have not complied with her requests. Prior to speaking to the resident, you have already begun to form an initial impression of behaviors which may be challenging for the team to manage—Ms. A presents as entitled and demanding, is pulling for increasingly more attention and involvement from medical staff, while also devaluing and engaging them with hostility. You anticipate that the primary team may be managing uncomfortable negative countertransference toward Ms. A, feeling ensnared in working up a serious medical conundrum while simultaneously being subjected to her splitting, anger, and seemingly relentless or unreasonable demands [19].

You call the primary team, and the resident explains that they have a high suspicion that Ms. A is surreptitiously injecting herself with insulin, intentionally causing the episodes of hypoglycemia. The team would like to discharge her; however, she has become dangerously hypoglycemic each time she has stabilized and learned that she was progressing toward leaving the hospital. They are concerned that Ms. A will continue to escalate, become aggressive, or harm herself if she is confronted with their suspicions, and are hoping that she can be psychiatrically hospitalized, making the case that "she is clearly a danger to herself."

You ask the resident about factors in Ms. A's hospital course that have prompted their concern for factitious disorder, as this diagnosis warrants both exclusion of an underlying medical condition *and* evidence supporting deception through symptom falsification [20]. Ms. A has had repeated hospital presentations with hypoglycemia without an identified cause, each one accompanied by multiple requests for additional unnecessary tests and inpatient hospitalization, which has now escalated in severity, likely to ensure hospitalization would be granted. She has been insisting—using unusually specific and sophisticated medical terminology—that adrenal insufficiency was identified at an outside hospital. She has refused to provide consent to allow access to her outside medical records, which is often imperative in identifying historical inconsistencies in factitious disorder [20]. The team has conducted a thorough workup based on their initial broad differential diagnosis for hypoglycemia—including hepatic and pituitary dysfunction, adrenal insufficiency, autoimmune disorders, infection, occult substance use, and autonomous insulin production from a functional tumor—none of which has identified an underlying medical etiology. Furthermore, the period of sustained normoglycemia after Ms. A was relocated to the MICU and under a higher level of observation suggested a potential self-induced mechanism for her symptoms. With growing suspicions, the team measured Ms. A's blood glucose, serum insulin, proinsulin, and c-peptide concentrations during her third hypoglycemic episode. They found c-peptide to be suppressed, along with the presence of synthetic insulin, indicating exogenous insulin administration. Floor staff searched the patient's room while she was in radiology and did not find medication or paraphernalia but felt uncomfortable searching her belongings without consent. Given the potential for profound medical and psychological consequences from a misdiagnosis or premature discharge, the team has been cautious in excluding medical pathology and verifying their concerns, reaching the reasonable degree of certainty desired for making a factitious disorder diagnosis [20].

The medicine resident adds that the team and floor staff are eager to confront Ms. A about their findings but are fearful that she may cause serious injury to herself if not also expeditiously discharged or moved to the monitored setting of an inpatient psychiatric unit. You recognize that the primary team's sense of urgency and "eagerness" behind the confrontation and discharge of Ms. A may relate to a desire to gratify the anger that they are experiencing, or to alleviate fear and anxiety related to the risk of the patient harming herself while under their care. Interactions with a patient with factitious disorder can be unintentionally influenced by frustration, anger and a drive for retribution—to hold her accountable for the deception and manipulation in which she has been "caught." The team may feel duped, injured, and that their empathy and trust have been exploited; this can be accompanied by feelings of being *stuck*, held hostage in caring for a deceptive patient who remains medically vulnerable and in need of treatment.

The role for the psychiatric consultant in cases of suspected factitious disorder is manifold: to assess for psychiatric comorbidity and suicidality, to ensure safe and effective hospital care and disposition, to assist the primary team in managing any other challenging behaviors that interfere with care, and to aid in managing countertransference issues. Patients with factitious disorder have higher rates of comorbid personality disorders, childhood physical and sexual abuse, and neglect [21, 22]. Thus, one important task of the psychiatrist is to help recognize acting out behaviors from the patient and to assist in mitigating related enactments—i.e., the unconscious repetition of early hostile or neglectful relationships with caregivers—that can occur between the challenging patient and her providers. As a first step, you arrange for a meeting with the primary team and nursing staff to plan your collective approach to Ms. A and discuss how the team can ensure safety as she receives ongoing care in the hospital and during the discharge process.

You meet with the primary team and begin the process of addressing countertransference through explicit acknowledgement of the shared frustration, anger, and fear you anticipate they might be experiencing, along with provision of psychoeducation to address misconceptions and support their remaining empathy for the patient. You highlight that factitious disorder typically involves the conscious fabrication of illness, but with an unconsciously motivated need to be in the sick role with its component closeness and receipt of caring attention. You contrast this psychiatric diagnosis with malingering, which is consciously motivated by the desire for external rewards (i.e., secondary gain) [3]. You note that patients with factitious disorder often have experienced illness, trauma, and loss in childhood. This history may be associated with a preoccupation with medical care, higher rates of comorbid depression, substance use, and character pathology, as well as underlying illness anxiety contributing to their symptom fabrication and care-seeking. You emphasize the probability that the patient is acting out of distress, rather an overt or conscious desire to fool and manipulate the medical team [19, 21, 22]. Together, you weigh the potential risks and benefits of confronting Ms. A and decide that it is a necessary intervention given her active and high-risk attempts to perpetuate illness and hospitalization. Existing evidence supports the presence of the consulting psychiatrist in therapeutic confrontations for patients with factitious disorder. This helps to provide support to both the team and the patient, communicate a consistent and unified message to the patient (thus reducing the risk for splitting), and will allow the consultant to begin the process of assessing the patient psychiatrically [19]. You outline the elements of an optimal approach to patients with factitious disorder and join the team as they meet with Ms. A.

You find Ms. A alone in her room, and she begins to detail various symptoms she is experiencing immediately after the primary team greets her. You introduce yourself and your role on the team, and her demeanor changes as she appears alarmed and becomes quiet. The primary attending proceeds to present Ms. A with the team's diagnostic impression, as recommended: allowing the patient to "save face" by avoiding critical and accusatory language or pressing the patient for an explanation or admission of responsibility. The primary attending conveys an empathic understanding that the patient is clearly in distress, while also communicating firmly that no further testing is indicated in the hospital. However, the attending is also careful to stress to Ms. A that she will continue to receive the care she needs while in the hospital and as an outpatient following her discharge [19, 22, 23]. You add that one aspect of providing the patient with the optimal care that she "deserves" is ensuring that she is safe while in the hospital and that she receives appropriate support and treatment after she leaves. While Ms. A listens intently, she is irritable and adamantly denies playing a role in inducing hypoglycemia.

You remain in the room with Ms. A after the team departs to provide support and continue your evaluation. You make efforts to build rapport by focusing on the distress she may be experiencing, as well as your desire to identify and provide the emotional care that she may need [22]. Ms. A initially remains guarded and superficial, returning repeatedly and defensively to denying use of exogenous insulin without your prompting. Ms. A denies all psychiatric symptoms and suicidal ideation as you assess for comorbidities, and you gently broaden the scope of the interview, inquiring into her life outside of the hospital in order to better contextualize her presentation. You learn that she is an emergency department nurse who works two jobs to support her children and is in the process of separating from her husband. Employment in healthcare and the presence of major psychosocial stressors are common factors in factitious disorder [19, 20], and you begin to frame these as possible contributors to Ms. A's psychological distress. She reluctantly agrees to accept a referral for psychotherapy, conceding that it would be helpful to have added support given the "stress" that she has been managing on her own. Although there is insufficient evidence for any specific psychiatric treatment modality for factitious disorder—in part due to the expectedly poor patient engagement in follow-up—you maintain hope that Ms. A will benefit from a long-term psychotherapeutic relationship that will facilitate gaining expanded insight into her behavior and motives, while providing supportive treatment [24].

You return to the primary team to debrief the therapeutic confrontation with Ms. A and to discuss a collaborative treatment plan for all team members to follow. Critically, you first recommend implementing close monitoring with one-to-one observation to ensure her safety while in the hospital, particularly as you anticipate potential for further behavioral escalation as the primary team begins the process of discharging her. You provide referrals for outpatient psychotherapy and explain to the team that there is no indication that inpatient psychiatric treatment has added benefit in the management of factitious disorder in the absence of psychiatric comorbidity [24]. You conclude the consultation by clearly documenting the interaction with Ms. A, charting her diagnosis and the evidence supporting it—which the team has been reluctant to do out of concern for making a potentially stigmatizing diagnosis, but is an essential process for informing clinicians involved in her care. This helps to ensure Ms. A's safety during her current and future hospitalizations and reduces the risk for iatrogenic harm [23]. You note your plan to continue to follow Ms. A for the duration of her hospitalization in an effort to provide ongoing assessment, as well as support for the patient and team. Aside from ensuring Ms. A's safety and assisting in connecting her to psychiatric treatment, remaining a present and involved consultant offers helpful reassurance for the medical team. Doing so provides an important opportunity to assist the team as they navigate other challenging behaviors and interpersonal dynamics that may arise, along with the intense countertransference issues that may be encountered while continuing to deliver care to a patient with factitious disorder.

Appendix: Summary Table

	Problems	Strategies
• Patient symptoms and behaviors	• Presence of somatic symptoms without identified medical etiology • Illness anxiety and distress related to somatic symptoms • Shifting or escalating physical complaints • Deceptive behaviors ranging from symptom exaggeration to symptom fabrication	• Assess for psychiatric comorbidities and recommend specific pharmacologic and psychotherapeutic treatment when appropriate • Assess for psychosocial stressors, consider presence of secondary gain, collaborate with social work and offer resources to address concrete stressors • Provide empathic support or tactful confrontation of deceptive behaviors, remain non-critical, and allow patient to "save face" when confrontation is necessary; consider increased observation levels to ensure safety [22, 23] • Assess for underlying illness anxiety in cases of symptom exaggeration
• Provider-patient dynamics	• Patient has dependent or histrionic personality traits interfering with care or creating provider distress • Patient frequently seeking reassurance from provider or is demanding increased or unnecessary care • Provider frustrated, hopeless, and is avoiding a demanding patient with medically unexplained symptoms	• Mitigate provider avoidance and patient anxiety by encouraging team to schedule regular, consistent meetings with the patient (e.g., once or twice daily immediately following rounds) • Encourage team to offer empathic reassurance to the patient using clear and direct language, referencing objective evidence from workup; resist the temptation to pursue or satisfy every patient concern and request if not medically indicated; set and maintain clear and reasonable limits on provider time and availability • Reassure the patient regarding the consistency of care and the role for ongoing outpatient medical follow-up and support; provide written information or other tangible aids regarding relevant symptoms and diagnoses as the patient approaches transitions in their care [15]

(continued)

	Problems	Strategies
• Inter-provider and provider-family dynamics	• Provider identifies somatic or functional symptoms as entirely "psychological" and wishes to transition treatment to psychiatry • Family rejecting of team's impression of functional or factitious symptoms, family is confused, or angry and devaluing in response	• Provide psychoeducation regarding the role of psychiatry and ongoing medical follow-up, partner with the primary team and highlight the need for close collaboration between medical and psychiatric providers • Re-engage providers with additional workup only when indicated, or provide specific active interventions to be made (e.g., involving physical therapy in recovery from functional neurological symptoms) • Encourage family support in the care of the patient, elicit patient and family views on illness and patient symptoms; provide psychoeducation regarding reciprocal relationship between psychosocial difficulties and physical symptoms; validate concerns, familial and patient distress, and link to the utility of psychiatric treatment [10, 15]
• Patient-provider barriers	• Mismatch between patient and provider treatment goals • Patient requests for testing or treatment that is not indicated • Patient refusal of psychiatric consultation and referral	• Focus on the "common ground" by acknowledging and addressing patient distress related to symptoms • Offer clear, unambiguous, and reassuring explanations for why a test or treatment is not indicated; emphasize shared desire to minimize risk for iatrogenic harm or side effects • Counsel primary team on tactful, supportive strategies for presenting diagnostic impressions; educate patient on the role of psychiatric treatment as collaborative with ongoing medical care; focus on the patient's experience of symptoms and coping with them; avoid language that might be experienced as invalidating, or a premature focus on the psychological etiologies of patient symptoms; provide education on evidence-based role for antidepressant medications and psychotherapy in addressing certain medical symptoms (e.g., chronic pain) [15]

• Hospital system barriers	• Multiple medical symptoms and specialist consultations resulting in fragmented and redundant care • Patient makes threats of litigation, suicide contingent on discharge • Limited access to outside medical records	• Ensure patient has a primary care physician who will be "steering the ship" and can consolidate treatment to the minimum number of physicians and clinical systems possible, avoid redundant testing to appease patient • Encourage involvement of legal department, hospital administration, ethics consultations as indicated [23] • Clearly document pertinent interactions with the patient, suicide risk assessment, clinical decision-making, and all diagnoses that are made during the hospitalization [23] • Utilize trusted sources of collateral information close to the patient, when contact information and consent is available; highlight the benefit of integrating psychiatric care, as well as outside sources of support and collateral information for optimizing the patient's treatment

References

1. Croicu C, Chwastiak L, Katon W. Approach to the patient with multiple somatic symptoms. Med Clin N Am. 2014;98:1079–95.
2. Henningsen P. Management of somatic symptom disorder. Dialogues Clin Neurosci. 2018;20:23–31.
3. American Psychiatric Association. Somatic symptom and related disorders. In: Diagnostic and statistical manual of mental disorders, vol. 5. Arlington: American Psychiatric Association; 2013.
4. Kleinstäuber M, Witthöft M, Steffanowski A, van Marwijk H, Hiller W, Lambert M. Pharmacological interventions for somatoform disorders in adults. Cochrane Database Syst Rev. 2014;(11):CD010628.
5. van Dessel N, den Boeft M, van der Wouden JC, Kleinstäuber M, Leone SS, Terluin B, et al. Non-pharmacological interventions for somatoform disorders and medically unexplained physical symptoms (MUPS) in adults. Cochrane Database Syst Rev. 2014;(11):CD011142.
6. Abbass A, Kisely S, Kroenke K. Short-term psychodynamic psychotherapy for somatic disorders. Psychother Psychosom. 2009;78:265–74.
7. Maunder RG, Hunter JJ, Atkinson L, Steiner M, Wazana A, Fleming AS. An attachment-based model of the relationship between childhood adversity and somatization in children and adults. Psychosom Med. 2017;79:506–13.
8. Mellers J. The approach to patients with "non-epileptic seizures". Postgrad Med J. 2005;81:498–504.
9. Asadi-Pooya ASS. Psychogenic nonepileptic seizures: a concise review. Neurol Sci. 2017;38:935–40.
10. Stone J. Functional symptoms and signs in neurology: assessment and diagnosis. J Neurol Neurosurg Psychiatry. 2005;76:i2–i12.
11. Avbersek A, Sisodiya S. Does the primary literature provide support for clinical signs used to distinguish psychogenic nonepileptic seizures from epileptic seizures? J Neurol Neurosurg Psychiatry. 2010;81:719–25.
12. Jones B, de Williams AC. CBT to reduce healthcare use for medically unexplained symptoms: systematic review and meta-analysis. Br J Gen Pract. 2019;69:e262–9.
13. McKenzie P, Oto M, Russell A, Pelosi A, Duncan R. Early outcomes and predictors in 260 patients with psychogenic nonepileptic attacks. Neurology. 2009;74:64–9.
14. Carton S, Thompson PJ, Duncan JS. Non-epileptic seizures: patients' understanding and reaction to the diagnosis and impact on outcome. Seizure. 2003;12:287–94.
15. Stone J. Functional symptoms in neurology: management. J Neurol Neurosurg Psychiatry. 2005;76:i13–21.
16. Stone J, Binzer M, Sharpe M. Illness beliefs and locus of control. J Psychosom Res. 2004;57:541–7.

17. LaFrance WC, Baird GL, Barry JJ, Blum AS, Frank Webb A, Keitner GI. Multicenter pilot treatment trial for psychogenic nonepileptic seizures. JAMA Psychiatr. 2014;71:997.
18. Hinson VK, Weinstein S, Bernard B, Leurgans SE, Goetz CG. Single-blind clinical trial of psychotherapy for treatment of psychogenic movement disorders. Parkinsonism Relat Disord. 2006;12:177–80.
19. Reich P, Gottfried LA. Factitious disorders in a teaching hospital. Ann Intern Med. 1983;99:240–7.
20. Krahn LE, Li H, O'Connor MK. Patients who strive to be ill: factitious disorder with physical symptoms. Am J Psychiatry. 2003;160:1163–8.
21. Yates GP, Feldman MD. Factitious disorder: a systematic review of 455 cases in the professional literature. Gen Hosp Psychiatry. 2016;41:20–8.
22. Bass C, Halligan P. Factitious disorders and malingering: challenges for clinical assessment and management. Lancet. 2014;383:1422–32.
23. Taylor JB, Beach SR, Kontos N. The therapeutic discharge: an approach to dealing with deceptive patients. Gen Hosp Psychiatry. 2017;46:74–8.
24. Eastwood S, Bisson JI. Management of factitious disorders: a systematic review. Psychother Psychosom. 2008;77:209–18.

Malingering

9

Rachel Knight and Christina Shayevitz

Your pager reads: "The patient is pulling out her lines and yelling at staff – can you sedate her?"

The question is stated in an urgent manner, communicating that the patient's agitation requires an immediate response by the consult team. Agitation can quickly escalate to aggression that can compromise the safety of the patient and the team, as well as the ability to deliver necessary care. This *pager question* should be treated as urgent until clarified further, and a quick response—beginning with prompt verbal communication with the primary team—is important. The *consult* should be considered urgent if the patient's behavior is described as being within a spectrum between intense emotional arousal with motor restlessness, and threatening or violent actions endangering self or staff and compromising medical care. This may require immediate intervention with medications or brief use of restraints to ensure the safety of the patient and providers.

Once you determine the urgency of the consult and address immediate safety issues, there will be further layers of this consult request to begin to examine. This can be accomplished by clarifying the team's request to "sedate" the patient. This request com-

R. Knight (✉) · C. Shayevitz
Department of Psychiatry, NewYork-Presbyterian Hospital/
Weill Cornell Medicine, New York, NY, USA
e-mail: rnk9002@med.cornell.edu

A. Gorun et al. (eds.), *The Psychiatric Consult*,
https://doi.org/10.1007/978-3-031-26837-3_9

municates a need to manage problematic behavior, but the question to elaborate is, *why*? Is the team feeling exhausted or exasperated from having to respond to the patient's behavioral outbursts multiple times per day? Is the agitation provoking fear and avoidance, or interfering with the team's ability to provide important and potentially life-saving treatment?

Agitation management can often lead to a separation of service, wherein psychiatry is relied upon for pharmacological or restraint recommendations to address the patient's behavior, while the primary team continues to focus on the patient's medical needs. While this can be a critical part of the management strategy, the psychiatric consultant should also work to clarify the origin of the patient's agitation, inspire empathic understanding among those caring for the patient, and create collaborative strategies to prevent future escalation, in an effort to improve the care and outcomes for the patient.

Clinical Scenario

You call the primary team and ask the resident if the patient is currently agitated and if there are active safety concerns. The resident does not think so but admits he has not seen the patient yet, because he has been busy with other tasks. He has been receiving numerous pages from the nurse about the patient becoming increasingly agitated. He says that the patient has been "giving everyone trouble," and he questions if the patient should have been admitted to the hospital in the first place.

You ask the resident to tell you about the circumstances of the patient's admission and **hospital** course. He tells you that the patient, Ms. A, is a woman in her early 40s who presented to the emergency department complaining of nonspecific back pain. During the initial interview, she had seemed annoyed by questions and did not provide the admitting team with much meaningful history. She did specifically ask to be admitted to the hospital for "pain control," despite not outwardly appearing to the admitting team to be in significant pain.

You reviewed the outpatient records which revealed that Ms. A has a history of multiple myeloma. She attended only a few of the oncology appointments scheduled for her and had stopped following up for chemotherapy months ago. The office staff had been trying to reach Ms. A without success, and it seems she had "fallen off of everyone's radar" following multiple canceled and missed appointments. There is no information in the chart about her living situation or social supports. Although Ms. A did not objectively appear to be in distress in the emergency room and her initial workup was normal, she was admitted to the medical service to rule out disease progression or sequelae, given her chief complaint of back pain in the setting of poor follow-up with her oncologist, and nonadherence with cancer treatment.

While you and the resident are speaking, the resident is paged by the nurse caring for Ms. A. The patient had just pulled out her intravenous (IV) line and is refusing for it to be replaced. The resident asks, "Can you come assess the patient now and sedate her?" He tells you that Ms. A needs this IV line for an MRI with contrast and that transport staff are on their way to pick her up. He adds, "If we can't get the IV in or make her stay still, she can't get the MRI, and it is the only thing holding up her discharge." The resident also mentions how burdensome it would be to have to reschedule the MRI and to keep her in the hospital for another day.

Scenario 1: Malingering and Medical Illness

You decide to see the patient right away and meet the resident in the nurses' station. He tells you he has tried several times to engage Ms. A in a discussion about her care. She knows she has "some type of cancer" but is uninterested in learning more about what this may mean for her and what treatment options are available. Instead, she interrupts bedside rounds and is preoccupied with asking for extra meal trays and snacks. She is described as malodorous and having signs of environmental exposure, suggesting that she may be homeless. Ms. A seems content as long as no one bothers her and she has access to food, and the resident suspects she is using the hospital for secondary gain, such as food and shelter (see Tables 9.1 and 9.2 for common forms of secondary gain and clues for when to suspect malingering). The resident tells you, "It's like

Table 9.1 Common forms of secondary gain in the hospital setting (i.e., external motivators)

• Temporary food or shelter
• Missing work
• Avoiding other unwanted duties (jail sentence, military service)
• Obtain drugs
• Obtain financial compensation
• Personal injury or disability claims

Table 9.2 When to suspect malingering

• Atypical presentation of chief complaint
• Rare symptoms
• Improbable symptoms
• Symptom combinations that rarely occur together
• Historical report of unusual responses to treatment/interventions
• Suspicion of tangible external incentives (i.e., an individual who is homeless presenting in context of extreme weather)
• Suspicion of voluntary control over symptoms
• Marked discrepancy between the reported symptoms and objective findings

she doesn't even care that she has cancer." He tells you more about her diagnosis and that the right treatment could possibly result in disease remission. He seems frustrated while describing this and mentions "I have a lot of patients who are scared to death about their diagnosis and would give anything for treatment options, and all she seems to care about is her next meal." You start to speculate that the resident is feeling exhausted and perhaps resentful, as if he is investing more effort into the patient's illness and treatment than she is. It seems like he is genuinely trying hard to treat what he identifies as her primary problem, the cancer. However, the suspicion for malingering—based on the patient's seeming lack of concern for her illness—has contributed to his generally negative countertransference toward Ms. A.

You suddenly hear yelling coming from the patient's room and enter to find Ms. A swinging her arm at the nurse who is attempting to replace an IV line. She is screaming "Get away from me! I don't need that!" The nurse looks frustrated and steps back to allow the resident speak. The resident explains, “We talked about this already, Ms. A. You need an IV so that contrast can be administered for the MRI.” Ms. A interrupts, “I don’t need an MRI, I’ve had one of those already!” The resident sighs and says, “Like I’ve explained before, you had an MRI years ago, but you need another one now so that we can figure out what is causing your pain, and to assess for disease progression.” The nurse looks at you from across the bedside and says “I don’t feel comfortable replacing the IV unless you give her something to calm her down.” Hearing this, the patient sits up in bed, glares at the nurse, and screams “I don’t need help to calm down, as long as you stay away from me with that needle! I’m planning on leaving here tomorrow anyway.” The nurse makes an expression of exasperation as she leaves the room, mumbling to the resident about having to cancel transportation and delay the MRI again.

You start to feel anxious and confused and realize that this may provide a clue into what is happening between Ms. A and the medical team. Ms. A seems upset while the team seems eager to quiet her. Through observation, you notice that there seem to be two separate conversations occurring in parallel: the patient’s goals are clearly different from those of her medical providers, and the discrepancy is causing mutual misunderstanding and conflict.

You return to Ms. A’s room to talk to her alone and bring with you some snacks that you found in the kitchen. She seems pleased with this, begins to calm, and allows you to ask her questions. You learn that she has very little understanding about her cancer diagnosis and the potential treatment options. She remembers being told previously that she had cancer but was surprised to learn about the diagnosis and still questions it, noting that “I feel fine, why would I need treatment?” She goes on to explain, “I’ve got enough to worry about, so why worry about something that isn’t bothering me?” You ask her about the things that are worrying her and learn that she is intermittently homeless and lives month-to-month off of her social security checks. She typically gets by on this alone, but this month she left her shelter because she felt unsafe after her clothing and food stamps were stolen. She used what was left of her income to purchase a new jacket and buy food and had no money left over and no place to stay for the last 2 days of the month. Ms. A planned to come into the hospital just until the first of the month, when she is eligible to pick up her next check.

You realize that both the patient and her medical team share a focus on her well-being and "survival"; however, both seem to have very different priorities and ideas of what that means. The medical team knows that the patient may die if her cancer is not adequately treated. They identify a problem that they have the training and expertise to help address, but the patient is behaving in a way that interferes with that help. Meanwhile, Ms. A is struggling to meet her basic needs and is not in a position to focus on what her team considers to be her primary issue. You ask Ms. A if she would be willing to stay in the hospital longer and allow for the necessary medical workup if the team were also able to enlist social work support to explore other options to help meet her other needs. Ms. A agrees and seems to find reassurance in hearing that some of her concerns outside of the hospital are also being acknowledged and prioritized.

You find the medical team and help them to devise strategies for working with the patient. While it is true that Ms. A is technically malingering given her external incentive to use the hospital for food and shelter, you explain that this is an adaptive survival strategy. You express understanding that it must feel difficult to treat a patient who seems to be indifferent to her own medical care but wonder if it may help to elicit empathy by sharing your understanding that Ms. A has had to worry about feeling safe at night and meeting her other basic, immediate needs. You suggest that the team make efforts to also focus on the social determinants of health that are limiting the patient's ability to engage in healthcare by utilizing the team social worker, who has knowledge of resources that may be helpful to the patient (see *Summary Table* for an outline of social determinants of health and ways to utilize outpatient resources). Bolstering Ms. A's access to critical resources and making efforts to address the concerns she identifies as her priority outside of the hospital may help her to feel understood and supported and to better engage in her own healthcare.

In this scenario, the patient presented reporting severe pain which has been incongruent with her exam and the medical team's clinical observations and is now avoiding the necessary medical workup that they have recommended. Malingering is often considered when there is suspicion for false or exaggerated symptoms with identifiable external motivation. This scenario highlights an important consideration, which is that malingering is not an *absolute* condition—malingering patients may also have true comorbid mental or medical illnesses and are in need of treatment and compassionate care. As the consulting psychiatrist, you are in a unique position to help the team navigate the necessary treatment of a patient who is otherwise labeled as being *manipulative* or *difficult*. By thoroughly exploring the patient's motives and priorities, you can help the team to reframe the way they think about and interact with the patient and potentially improve the way the patient navigates and engages with medical treatment in the future.

Scenario 2: Malingering in a Patient Who Uses Substances

You return the page from the medical team and learn that the patient has been escorted down to the MRI suite twice already earlier in the day. The scan was terminated early on both attempts when Ms. A yelled out in pain and refused to continue. She has been telling the primary team that she needs stronger pain medication in order to tolerate laying down and remaining still for an extended period of time. The resident tells you that the patient came in with track marks on her extremities and endorsed using intravenous heroin. He notes that, for this reason, the team is trying to limit the amount of pain medication she is given and is avoiding opioids altogether so as not to "reinforce her addiction." The resident goes on to say that Ms. A is "obviously *just* trying to get us to give her opioids," and he is hoping to have you recommend something to "sedate her" in order to get the necessary imaging completed.

You pick up on the resident's frustration—and consider the potential impact of biases against patients with substance use disorders—in the assumption that Ms. A is trying to manipulate him into prescribing higher doses of pain medication. It is easy for you to relate to his frustration. You are well aware that even in your own field of psychiatry, attitudes toward individuals with co-occurring substance use disorders are more negative than are attitudes toward individuals with other mental illnesses [1]. These attitudes are often colored by past negative experiences caring for individuals with substance use disorders and feelings of hopelessness for this particularly challenging-to-treat patient population, who also tend to have a poorer prognosis and greater illness severity. You know that stigmatizing and negative attitudes can lead to undertreatment, poorer communication, and worsening psychological distress for the hospitalized patient. These patients are vulnerable to feeling unheard when they speak out about being in pain, which can lead to a crisis of trust between the patient and their medical team. You formulate that your approach must be one that validates the patient's need for pain control while partnering with her to strengthen motivation for both medical and substance abuse treatment.

When you interview Ms. A, you acknowledge and empathize with the pain she is experiencing. You introduce your role as the consulting psychiatrist and tell the patient that you intend to help formulate a plan to keep her comfortable while she receives necessary medical attention. She has a very limited understanding of why the team is so worried about progression of disease and why she needs another MRI. Ms. A reiterates that she already had an MRI a few years ago and therefore should not need another. You take a substance use history and learn the patient is an active IV heroin user and currently uses up to 20 bags of heroin per day. She was previously enrolled in a methadone program and says her dose was 80 milligrams (mg) daily. You take note of this—80 mg is a high dose and it may reflect the patient's attempt to present herself as someone who needs higher doses of opioids while in hospital. However, if true, it can also mean that the patient has a severe opioid use disorder, may have a higher tolerance to pain medication, and will require a robust pain management regimen. The patient seems irritable and short-tempered with you throughout the interview. She interrupts frequently and uses a harsh and devaluing tone at times; she has insight into this and catches herself, apologizing frequently as if she is having trouble controlling her behavior. Ms. A notes that she has been experiencing withdrawal symptoms for hours and is tired of feeling judged by the treatment team whenever she asks for more medication. She tells you that she pulled out her IV line in an attempt to leave the hospital in order to use heroin, noting "If the doctors aren't going to treat my pain, I'll have to take care of it myself."

After leaving the patient, you call her methadone clinic and confirm that her past dose was indeed 80 mg per day. You reference a controlled substance registry and do not see that she is receiving any other controlled prescription medications. In this scenario, it is important to recognize and reflect on your own feelings toward the patient. Her tone and irritability made you feel frustrated and devalued, but her apparent insight into her behavior and her acknowledgement of it being impulsive and uncharacteristic of her helped to mitigate these feelings. You conceptualize her as someone whose agitation is multifactorial: she has a severe opioid use disorder and is in withdrawal, she is experiencing undertreated pain, and she also may have limited affect regulation, frustration tolerance, and coping skills at her baseline. You begin to reframe her substance use as perhaps a maladaptive attempt to attenuate both physical and psychological pain and distress. Additionally, you consider that a low level of health literacy may be contributing to her continued poor understanding of her medical condition, despite multiple explanations from her medical team.

Strategies for the team to use as they approach Ms. A should focus on finding a balance between healthy skepticism and making sure the patient feels validated, understood, and cared for. Direct confrontation with suspicions of malingering for medication should be avoided, as it may alienate a patient in need of care, pain control, and treatment engagement. There is evidence that Ms. A likely has developed opioid dependence and tolerance, as well as increased pain sensitivity from chronic opioid use. Since Ms. A may also have acute back pain from her comorbid medical condition, you recommend that the medical team consider a pain management consultation to assist in optimizing pain control and to ensure that the patient's primary concern is being acknowledged and actively addressed. In addition, you can evaluate for and treat withdrawal symptoms as well as commonly co-occurring psychiatric disorders (e.g., anxiety, mood, and trauma-related disorders), which may be reciprocally impacting the patient's experience of pain and difficulty tolerating distress in the hospital.

Lastly, given the patient's poor health literacy, you counsel the primary team on using a modified communication style. You offer guidance around simplifying the medical jargon and breaking down complex information to be more clear, consistent, understandable, and patient-centered when discussing the specifics of her care. Improved communication, patient understanding of illness, and the alliance between the patient and her providers are critical to optimizing treatment adherence.

Scenario 3: Malingering and Primitive Defenses

You gather more information from the primary resident and learn about the patient's social situation. Ms. A is an unmarried mother of three adult children and currently lives alone. Her children have visited her on occasion throughout her hospitalization. They bring her food or flowers and seem to be positively involved in her life. However, the resident also notes that on several occasions staff members have had to intervene after hearing angry yelling coming from Ms. A's hospital room during these visits.

The medical resident tells you that there have been multiple attempts to perform an MRI, but the patient has refused each time for various vague and inconsistent reasons. On one attempt, for example, Ms. A refused to have the MRI done until her son arrived to accompany her. Ms. A subsequently refused to go after her son arrived, claiming that he was only able to visit for a short time and she didn't want to miss spending it with him. The resident tells you that Ms. A has been "difficult" to provide care for, and he can't understand why she seems intent on delaying her medical workup. He elaborates that Ms. A is typically very charismatic and friendly but is often challenging to interact with on rounds as she inevitably steers the conversation away from her medical care in favor of seemingly irrelevant topics. The resident finds it difficult to redirect or disengage from these discussions and to leave her room, as she often begs for him to stay "just a little longer." He also notes a "different side to her" and says it seems like her personality changes abruptly, and she seems to become angry about having more testing done. She will suddenly adopt a hostile tone and scream at the team in an unpredictable manner, especially as the team has attempted to move her care forward. The primary team is concerned that she may have significant progression of disease, and the MRI is a necessary next step in her workup. The resident is worried that talking with Ms. A again about the importance of the MRI will "get us nowhere" and wants you to provide recommendations for sedating her, so that the team can finally continue the medical workup.

When you arrive at the patient's room, she welcomes you and seems to be happy to have a visitor. She tells you that she "has been through so much" and believes a psychiatrist would find her story to be very interesting. She agrees to talk with you, but first asks you to help her rearrange items around her room, and asks if you can get her some water and food before she continues. You try to attend to her comfort and have a sense of wanting to accommodate her requests. When you return with water you see she has struck up a conversation with the nutritionist and motions for you to pull up a chair and join the conversation. She introduces you to the nutritionist as "her psychiatrist" and asks if the two of you can "collaborate on [her] complicated case." You notice yourself feeling irritated but also wanting to remain friendly and well-liked—the patient is already speaking so kindly of you, and you find yourself wanting to meet the flattering expectations she seems to have. You also feel cautious of how quickly the patient has taken a liking to you—before you have had the chance to learn anything about her—as well as impatient, knowing you have several other consults to complete. You glance at your watch, cognizant of your limited time, and ask the patient if perhaps you can come back later when she and the nutritionist have finished meeting. The patient immediately becomes effusively apologetic and begs you not to leave just yet. She is eager to talk to you, but you can't help but feel frustrated by the amount of time you have spent in her room, with such little information being exchanged.

Ms. A eventually begins to tell you a detailed narrative of her life, and does so with dramatic flair. She painstakingly and repeatedly highlights the hardships she has overcome, including raising three children on her own after her husband "abandoned [her]." You ask Ms. A about her children; her affect brightens, and she tells you how wonderful and accomplished each one is. At other times in your discussion, she depicts them as ungrateful and unappreciative of all that she has sacrificed for them. You learn that Ms. A has been largely estranged from her children, who seem to resurface when she is in crisis and in need of their help. The last time she was hospitalized she was diagnosed with cancer. At that time, her children—whom she had not been in contact with for years—rallied around her and visited the hospital daily. Once Ms. A was discharged following that hospitalization, her children initially stopped by her house frequently to provide support, but their visits abruptly stopped seemingly "out of the blue." She goes on to speak at length about her feelings of being chronically underappreciated and abandoned by all those she cares about. You look at the clock and realize you have been sitting at Ms. A's bedside for nearly an hour. You feel anxious about needing to meet the rest of the consultation team for rounds in a few minutes but feel trapped. You tactfully try to interrupt her story and tell her that you must come back at a later time to finish your interview.

On rounds with your attending, you run into two of Ms. A's children in the hallway near her room. They appear exhausted. You gather collateral, and they tell a different story than what the patient had relayed to you earlier. They describe their mother as having a longstanding pattern of behaving dramatically and "manipulating" others for attention. It was hard for her to meet her children's emotional needs, as it always seemed she was focused primarily on her own. As adults, she has frequently oscillated between telling the children how wonderful they are and growing easily irritated, wounded, and resentful over trivial perceived slights. Arguments usually end in Ms. A crying, claiming that no one cares about her. Ms. A's children eventually started to distance themselves from her as they grew older and invested in their own families, and she has become increasingly isolated from them. When Ms. A was diagnosed with cancer, her children made an initial effort to support her as much as possible. However, when she started responding to chemotherapy and improving medically, she reverted to her old behavioral patterns and began accusing the children of not being present enough, neglecting to recognize or consider their needs. This time around, Ms. A's family is suspicious that she may have stopped attending her outpatient chemotherapy appointments, perhaps even with the intent to elicit her children's attention. They are aware of the delays to Ms. A obtaining an MRI and believe she may also be intentionally creating these delays in effort to prolong the hospitalization.

Your attending suggests that you use this information as clinical data to help understand the psychosocial factors contributing to the patient's challenging behavior. You recall your own negative countertransference while meeting with Ms. A and remember feeling like she was treating your time as if it were inexhaustible, all while providing you with superficial gratitude and premature praise. You experienced tension between your feelings of irritation and a desire to align with and meet her early, idealized opinion of you. You were derailed from completing your necessary tasks in the consultation and felt pulled into providing her with more time and latitude in the interview than you typically might, nervous about becoming yet another uncaring person who wishes to abandon her.

Ms. A seems eager to meet with any member of the hospital staff in order to share her story and, however, also seems to keep interactions long-winded and superficial, with minimal discussion of her medical care. You think about the enactment you had been a part of and how it relates to what her children seem to have experienced for years. You speculate that Ms. A likely has a profound need to be close to others but is quick to lash out and to feel rejected—perhaps as an unconscious way of maintaining a "safe" distance, avoiding the potential realization of her underlying fears of being abandoned entirely. You imagine that being faced with a serious illness may have heightened Ms. A's fear of abandonment and may be causing her to unconsciously act in ways that appear needy, demanding, and contradictory and are complicating and prolonging her care. Unfortunately, in her case, her attempts to have her emotional needs met are maladaptive and self-defeating, as they are directly impacting her ability to engage in the necessary medical workup and treatment.

In this scenario, the patient's underlying personality style (including narcissistic, dependent, and histrionic traits) are impacting her ability to tolerate stressors related to her interpersonal relationships and medical care. The interpersonal dynamics her family describes seems to also be playing out with her medical team. The team is well-intentioned and wants to help Ms. A, but they also find it difficult to contain her and to disengage from her when it would be most productive to do so. They are feeling exhausted by her frequent demands for personal attention, combined with her rejection of the treatment plan and attempts to prolong her hospitalization. This, in turn, may lead to the team's wish to avoid Ms. A altogether and only confirms her expectation of rejection.

The consulting psychiatrist can intervene by identifying recurring, maladaptive interpersonal patterns and assist the team in interacting with this challenging patient in a way that still prioritizes her medical care. You explain that you understand the team's tendency toward avoidance, but this may be interpreted by the patient as abandonment and an aversion to her and result in less engagement with her care. You explain the importance of balancing reassurance with clear and consistent boundary setting. The patient needs to feel assured of the team's commitment to her care, while being reminded firmly and consistently of the limits to provider time and knowledge. It can be helpful to have a set time and agreed upon agenda for daily rounding, so that the patient can be reassured by the team's stable presence and availability, and the team can refer to the prioritized discussion points when time is limited. You help the team formulate strategies for interacting with the patient in a way that reduces overall distress and does not make the patient feel rejected (*see Summary Table*). You also offer to participate in a family meeting while Ms. A is in the hospital in an effort to facilitate effective communication and to help the family members to best support their mother while maintaining their own boundaries.

Appendix: Summary Table

	Problems	Strategies
• Patient symptoms and behaviors	• Subjective report of atypical or rare symptoms and/or suspicions of external incentives (see Table 9.1) • Irritability, affective lability, or agitation when confronted about inconsistencies or suspicion of malingering • Seemingly unexplained or unfounded complaints • Nonadherence to assessment or treatment	• Attempt to verify symptoms and circumstances, favoring a clarifying approach over a confrontational one, avoid direct accusations and allow patient to "save face" when possible • Always explore alternate reasons behind nonadherence using a psychosocial perspective • Utilize collateral information to supply evidence to support or refute history: Reports from family, friends, community members, or other clinicians who have treated patient in the past • In cases of suspected malingering for opioids or benzodiazepines, use controlled substance registries or other forms of objective verification (e.g., medical record, methadone clinic) • For agitation that is refractory to attempts at de-escalation, can utilize as-needed medications or restraints to maintain safety

(continued)

	Problems	Strategies
• Provider-patient dynamics	• Mutual distrust can develop if team suspects patient is malingering; patient may feel they are being abandoned or that their concerns are being invalidated • Patient's use of immature defenses (e.g., splitting, idealizing and devaluing, projection, projective identification, acting-out) may cause provider to feel frustrated, resentful, or deskilled and impotent • Persistent requests for pain medications can result in providers feeling annoyed and exploited, prompting restricting of analgesic medications, and patient feeling unheard, alienated, or accused of falsifying symptoms • Patient agitation and irritability is contributing to staff frustration and resentment over treating the patient	• Educate team as to how malingering patients can also have a psychiatric or medical illness, which are not mutually exclusive. Help team identify areas where they can help the patient beyond treating the medical illness alone • Validate and empathize with team frustrations, help them to identify countertransference, help identify barriers to care, and explore enactments • Schedule rounding or check-in times that happen predictably every day and for a defined amount of time. This way, the patient can be reassured and contained by a consistent presence and agenda and may feel less rejected when the team is unavailable • Formulate a pain management plan that identifies and meets the patient's unique needs, attending to substance use history, and possible dependence and tolerance. Request assistance from pain management and addiction psychiatry when appropriate • Identify and treat etiology of agitation while working with team on behavioral modifications and inspiring an empathic stance

• Inter-provider and provider-family dynamics	• Team's feelings of anger, frustration, hopelessness, and exhaustion can result in avoidance of patient • Team relying on consultant to re-define treatment relationship, repair alliance, or set boundaries • Family absent or minimally involved due to longstanding conflict	• Offer to round with the team as opposed to separately • Assist in facilitating or repairing open communication between patient and primary team • Utilize brief family-based interventions to provide psychoeducation, facilitate communication, empower family to set visit schedule and boundaries • Recommend other supportive interventions for patient and family (e.g., chaplain services, social work, referrals for continued psychiatric care)
• Patient-provider barriers	• Misalignment in patient and provider priorities or goals of care, both parties unable to understand the priorities of the other, leading to dissatisfaction and mistrust • Low levels of patient education and health literacy	• Counsel and encourage primary team to use language that can be easily understood by the patient and to consider any recommendations in the context of patient's unique social determinates of health
• Hospital system barriers	• Patient has barriers to proper follow-up, including unstable housing, transportation, financial barriers	• Elicit assistance from social work department to optimize outpatient support and reduce barriers, exploring alternative supportive or subsidized housing, meal delivery services, community support groups, exploring options for reduced fare transportation for appointments

References

1. Avery J. Attitudes toward individuals with mental illness and substance use disorders among resident physicians. Prim Care Companion CNS Disord. 2019;21(1):18m02382.

Further Reading

Groves JE. Taking care of the hateful patient. N Engl J Med. 1978;298(16): 883–7.

Levenson J. The American Psychiatric Association publishing textbook of psychosomatic medicine and consultation-liaison psychiatry. Washington, DC: American Psychiatric Association; 2019. Chapter 14.

The Suicidal Patient

10

Anne Clark-Raymond and Julie Penzner

Your pager reads: "The patient told me he's going to kill himself."

This page, while a statement, actually begs many questions of the consultant. Suicidality is a feature of many psychiatric disorders; suicidal statements in themselves must be carefully assessed for both content and context. The page has a tone of urgency and seems to ask: is my patient safe? How can I keep my patient safe? In order to complete a safety assessment, you will need to obtain a detailed account of what the patient said, to whom, when, and what historical and contextual variables are relevant. Has the patient done anything to harm himself? What, in particular, did he threaten to do? What is the status of the patient's medical condition? How has the patient responded thus far (medically and emotionally) to treatment and hospitalization? Perhaps more at the crux of this page: what do I *do* about this patient's wanting to kill himself? Patients' suicidality often frightens clinicians, particularly non-psychiatric teams who may feel unequipped, deskilled, or even threatened. They may find the patient a liability risk or feel that their own medical efforts have been thwarted.

A. Clark-Raymond (✉)
NewYork-Presbyterian Hospital/Weill Cornell Medicine,
New York, NY, USA

J. Penzner
Department of Psychiatry, Duke Regional Hospital, Durham, NC, USA

A. Gorun et al. (eds.), *The Psychiatric Consult*,
https://doi.org/10.1007/978-3-031-26837-3_10

Clinical Scenario

Following a brief review of the chart, you discover that the patient, Mr. J, is a 26-year-old man with a chronic and severe course of ulcerative colitis, who is admitted to the colorectal surgery service and is now recovering from a total proctocolectomy with ileostomy. Discharge home had been anticipated soon. When you call the team back, the surgical resident seems harried and tells you that this is an "urgent" consult, disclosing to you that Mr. J had expressed suicidal ideation. When you begin to ask more questions regarding the specifics of what Mr. J said, the resident is quick to tell you that she does not know any further details and laments that "he was almost ready for discharge! Can you come ASAP?" You inform the resident that you have further preparation to do prior to seeing the patient but instruct her to—in the meantime—place Mr. J on a one-to-one observation to ensure his safety.

Scenario 1: Major Depressive Episode

Further exploration of the surgical progress notes reveals that Mr. J underwent the extensive surgical procedure without complications. His postoperative course has progressed as expected. He has advanced his diet, required minimal pain medication, and learned from nursing how to care for his ostomy at home. However, you see an "event" note from the early morning hours that a patient care assistant had charted that Mr. J expressed "SI" to her overnight. The note contains no further details except that the assistant had notified nursing, who documented that she could not reach an MD, as the overnight resident had been called into a complicated emergency surgery. You feel immediately anxious reading that the patient had not been assessed for safety at all overnight. Has he already harmed himself? You also note feeling irritated that the team did not obtain advice sooner to put Mr. J on a one-to-one observation. You realize that your reactions to this consult may indeed be clues that the team is sharing these same feelings and reactions, which may help to explain their insistence that Mr. J be evaluated quickly.

There is frustration inherent in the resident's complaint that Mr. J's suicidality is delaying his discharge. Prior to now, Mr. J has been a model patient, with a textbook hospital course. It seems to you that the team is now frustrated that Mr. J is feeling suicidal, as if he has deliberately complicated his care and thwarted his discharge. A worthy question: why is Mr. J voicing suicidal ideation at this point in his hospitalization? An important aspect of evaluating a suicidal patient is not only an assessment of the patient's level of planning, intent, access to lethal means, and psychiatric history but also understanding the precipitating factors or triggering event, time of onset, and how and to whom the suicidal ideation was disclosed. Responses can provide clues to the severity of a patient's suicide risk, as well as to diagnosis, treatment, and disposition.

Fortunately, you received the consult first thing in the morning. After heading to the surgical floor, you are relieved to see that the patient care assistant who had documented the event note is still on the unit, about to head home after her shift. You introduce yourself and ask for details about her interaction with Mr. J. She tells you that she had brought Mr. J a pitcher of water that he had requested, asking him why he was still awake at that hour in the morning. Mr. J reported to her that he had terrible insomnia. While in the room, the assistant found a piece of paper on the floor, a letter Mr. J had written to his family, saying he plans to kill himself once discharged home, as he "can't take it anymore." Mr. J snatched the note from the assistant before she could read it in its entirety. You find the patient's primary nurse, who has cared for the patient for the majority of his admission. The nurse is quite surprised to learn of Mr. J's suicidal ideation, which he had never mentioned previously. During his admission, he was quiet and well-mannered. The nurse does note that the patient never has any visitors, despite seeming to be a likeable young man.

In meeting Mr. J, you introduce yourself as a member of the psychiatry team and inquire if Mr. J is aware as to why you were called. He answers quietly, "because they found what I was journaling." His affect is notably flat, as he describes having felt depressed for several years, feeling that his life and career prospects are limited by his ulcerative colitis symptoms. He found his symptoms "humiliating" and "disgusting" and thus did not disclose them to friends or coworkers, nor to family, not wanting to "burden" anyone. He describes having gradually stopped answering calls or texts, so that now his former friends rarely check in with him. He has been living alone since graduating from college, with limited contact with his parents. While he first started to isolate himself because of his painful ulcerative colitis symptoms, he says that now he simply doesn't feel like socializing. He reports initially having wanted to undergo surgery to try to improve his life, but that since hospitalization he's only felt bleaker. He began to have thoughts of suicide soon after his operation. He could not think of a way to complete suicide in the hospital but had planned to overdose on pain medications at home upon discharge. Mr. J says that he didn't want to let the team know how he was feeling, as he did not want them to intervene to prevent suicide. You suspect there may have been some ambivalence about help-seeking, given that Mr. J did leave his note in a discoverable place.

You share with Mr. J your impression that he is depressed and can be helped with psychiatric treatment. As you do with all patients you see, you use the Columbia-Suicide Severity Rating Scale (C-SSRS) [1] as an evidence-based means of evaluating Mr. J's suicide risk. You determine that he is at high risk for suicide given his level of intent and planning. You discuss with him the necessity of an inpatient psychiatric hospitalization, and after providing him more information, Mr. J consents to a voluntary admission.

The team expresses relief that you have solved the issue of disposition of their patient. However, when you speak to the resident later in the day, she expresses her disappointment that Mr. J was suicidal—both disappointed in Mr. J for not being "happy" with the successful outcome of the surgery and also disappointed in herself: in her inability to help Mr. J actually resume his life and functioning and in her failure to notice his depression, a condition she "knows about" from medical school. The team's concern for Mr. J, as evidenced by their feelings of urgency in requesting your assistance and expertise, speaks to their own feelings of worry about him and potentially their feelings of helplessness in treating him. The team may feel guilty for not having noticed signs of Mr. J's depression sooner, though you can empathize with the surgical team's limited time to engage with him, drawing upon your own experience on the surgical and medical floors and recalling how difficult it is to simply manage all of your patients' day-to-day *medical* responsibilities, let alone unmentioned psychiatric concerns. It may come as a disappointment to the team to have successfully surgically cured this man's chronic and severe case of ulcerative colitis but ultimately be unable to save his life.

Although unlikely that they would admit it, it is likely that the team, at least in part, feels angry at Mr. J for being suicidal and angry that he actively thwarted (or undid) their successful surgical treatment and discharge plan. Notably, suicide is often an angry and aggressive act on the patient's part. While patients direct those aggressive feelings toward themselves via suicide, their suicidal ideation may be thought to reflect a deep-seated anger toward others or toward their circumstances. For Mr. J, this could be reflected in his feelings of humiliation and disgust toward his disease. Suicidality thus represents a method of acting out aggression and rage in the only way that may feel accessible to the patient. In turn, while the aggression is directed inwardly, suicides do effectively cause harm and suffering to friends, family, and physicians and other medical caregivers, who are left to cope with the loss of the person and the fallout from their death. All of these factors may, in turn, help to explain the team's frustration with the patient that was noticeable from the moment you returned the page. In your liaison role, you speak with the surgical resident, to help her process these complicated feelings. She finds your validation of her ambivalence about being unable to truly "cure" Mr. J to be helpful, if a bit unexpected.

Scenario 2: Borderline Personality Disorder

You take a few minutes to review Mr. J's chart and see that, compared to the commonly terse surgical notes, the team's daily progress notes are quite detailed in describing complex and heated interactions with Mr. J. From the first postoperative day, the notes detail Mr. J's rage after he discovered that an ostomy had been created for him, despite his knowledge that this (a) might be necessary and (b) could be reversed later. Notes detail Mr. J advancing his diet prematurely to solids, leading to a need for nasogastric tube placement. Mr. J refused an assessment by physical therapy, prolonging his discharge planning, and insisted that he could not care for his ostomy at home. His care needs were found to be too minimal to qualify for visiting nurse services. Nursing notes detail Mr. J's numerous requests for pain medication before it is due and describe him pulling out his IV each time a pain medication is refused. This results in a delay of the medication he had initially requested to be administered.

Since the resident you'd spoken to on the phone did not know the details of Mr. J's suicidal statement, she passed the phone to the intern on the team. The intern describes to you in hushed tones how the attending, Dr. B, learned yesterday that Mr. J had posted scathing reviews of her on a major online platform. Subsequently, Dr. B declared to Mr. J that he would be discharged the next day given that he was medically stable. Mr. J argued that he did not feel able to care for himself at home, but Dr. B replied that "discharge would be happening whether [Mr. J] likes it or not." The intern—who describes always feeling like "the good guy" in the team's relationship with Mr. J—reports that this morning Mr. J threatened that if he were discharged today, he would kill himself. He then showed the intern several superficial cuts he had made to his inner forearm using a Swiss Army knife that was in his possession. The intern explains to you, "I thought I, at least, had a good relationship with Mr. J. I don't know how we're ever going to be able to discharge him now!".

Steeling yourself for a contentious patient interview and a mess of a liaison role, you enter Mr. J's room. His one-to-one sitter gives you a sympathetic smile. Mr. J sees you and immediately barks, "who are you?". You begin to introduce yourself but are soon interrupted by Mr. J, who glibly says, "I know why they sent you - it's because I said I'm going to kill myself if they discharge me, and I will. There's nothing you can do!". You attempt to ask Mr. J how he is feeling currently and what his understanding is of his treatment and discharge plan. He angrily lists his complaints to you as had been detailed in the surgical notes. He is difficult to redirect. You attempt to gather the specifics of Mr. J's suicidal ideation, but he only cryptically insists to you that he has attempted suicide before, and will do so again, and does not mind if you try to involuntarily hospitalize him on a psychiatric unit as he's "enjoyed" it previously. Mr. J begins to scream at you to get out of the room, and in order to not risk him escalating further, as well as out of concern for your own safety, you comply.

You retreat to the surgical residents' workroom, defeated and fuming. There, as luck would have it, you find the surgical resident, intern, attending, and social worker, all eating a late lunch. They inquire as to your impressions of the patient. Before you can respond, the social worker complains, "he's holding us hostage - we're unable to discharge him!". At that time, the intern receives a page for an extra dose of pain medication that Mr. J isn't yet due for. The resident scoffs and says, "we're not giving him anything! Not after what he said to me today!" She explains that earlier today, Mr. J made disparaging comments to her about her gender and race. The intern replies quietly that he feels badly for Mr. J, to which the attending shoots back angrily, "that's the problem! He's playing on your sympathy!". You can sense the fierce conflict in this team, between them and Mr. J, but also among the clinicians themselves. It seems that Mr. J has effectively split the team, dividing them in what should be their common approach and treatment.

While you feel pulled to validate the team's anger—even hatred—of this patient, you also feel cautious in "taking sides" with the team in vilifying Mr. J. Your countertransference (the anger you feel toward Mr. J) reminds you of a lecture you had as a second year resident about the different psychological defenses used by patients. You recall learning about projective identification, a defense commonly employed by patients whose personality is organized at a borderline level (which includes patients with borderline personality disorder, as well as some patients with narcissistic, histrionic, and antisocial personality disorders or traits). You recall that projective identification occurs when a patient's own emotions are effectively *projected* onto the recipients (in this case, the treatment team), and the recipients then personally *identify* with these unpleasant feelings and harbor them as their own, rather than being able to appreciate these feelings as stemming from the patient's own conflicts, emotions, and reactions [2]. You remember learning that projective identification is one of the most uncomfortable experiences for a provider. Furthermore, in addition to likely projective identification, Mr. J is also actively reinforcing the actual non-projected anger the team feels by devaluing them, discriminating against them, and giving the team now "just cause" to feel hateful toward him. You are not sure how much of this to share with the team, so excuse yourself and buy some time to think.

You reluctantly return again the next day to see Mr. J, who continues angrily outlining his grievances. You alter your approach, remarking to him that you notice how incredibly angry this process has caused him to be. He answers snidely, "you think so, Doc? Yes! My life sucks." Mr. J then goes on to detail for you how he finds his diagnosis of ulcerative colitis to be yet another insult to him, following his struggles with a lifelong learning disability, having been physically abused by his step-father, and unable to attend college due to his family's finances. He mentions being particularly upset now by the presence of his ostomy bag, which he sees as an outwardly visible sign of his inadequacies. You begin to feel empathy toward Mr. J and can now appreciate his angry and spiteful actions as reactions to his own feelings of rage, helplessness, and powerlessness.

You just discovered some information that is critical in understanding Mr. J's interactions with the team. Explaining to the team in general terms this aspect of Mr. J's psychology can go a long way toward helping them also begin to feel some empathy toward him. While you certainly cannot justify to the team Mr. J's actions, you can help the team to understand the therapeutic value in building rapport with Mr. J by empathizing with and validating his experience and concerns. You suggest to the team that all members round on Mr. J together to interrupt the splitting, so that the team can maintain the common goal of a safe discharge. You are clear with the team that resolution of Mr. J's "hostage-taking" via expressed suicidal ideation is most likely to occur through empathy; empathy is also the most likely course toward psychotherapy, which will likely improve his post-surgical prognosis and treatment adherence. You prepare the team for the encounter: they should be firm in their decision to discharge, give Mr. J room to disagree with their decision, and remain calm during the interaction even if Mr. J becomes angry. You encourage the team to be transparent with Mr. J when explaining their decision-making process, including explaining the limitations in implementing certain medical and nursing services that Mr. J desires. Ideally, transparency will reduce the likelihood of further escalation in Mr. J, who is likely highly attuned to any unexpressed anger or vindictiveness on the part of his team, fueling his aggression.

You reassess Mr. J's suicidal feelings. Mr. J states that he often wishes he weren't alive and that he cuts himself to relieve this distress. While he also thinks of suicide, Mr. J reports feeling conflicted, since he also desires an improved life (as evidenced by his proceeding with surgery), and fears dying. While it seems that Mr. J is at an increased risk of suicide, you believe this risk is *chronically* elevated, given what you have diagnosed as borderline personality disorder including non-suicidal self-injury. You also know that patients with a primary diagnosis of a borderline pathology typically do not benefit from acute inpatient hospitalizations, which paradoxically may reinforce the patient's maladaptive, help-seeking, and help-rejecting behaviors, without altering the level of acute risk. You make Mr. J appointments with a psychiatrist and psychotherapist affiliated with your hospital's collaborative care psychiatry clinic, to better bridge the gap between the patient's medical and psychiatric care. After providing a hand-off to the collaborative care team, you encourage them to consider a comprehensive dialectical-behavioral therapy program as an eventual disposition plan.

Scenario 3: Coping with Medical Complications

In reviewing Mr. J's chart, you notice that it is extensive, with several postoperative notes describing multiple complications, including a surgical site infection requiring wound vacuum placement. Mr. J had also contracted a hospital-acquired infection and has required intravenous antibiotics, which has further delayed his recovery. Due to these complications, Mr. J's discharge planning has included going home with a peripherally inserted central catheter (PICC) line and frequent outpatient visits for wound vacuum changes.

You page the team back, hoping this will be a better time to gather information from them since their morning rounds have now ended. The intern returns your page and tells you that yesterday, while the nursing staff trained Mr. J to care for his ostomy, he voiced his lack of motivation about doing this at home, claiming "if this is what I have to do, I might as well just kill myself." The social worker on the team had similarly reported to the intern that in discussing with Mr. J the need for visiting nurse services to administer the antibiotics via his PICC line, he lamented, "just kill me now." The intern says to you that she's not surprised Mr. J has made these statements, as he's acted quite frustrated with each complication of his long hospital course. He's often irritable with the team and also his wife, who is regularly at his bedside in the evenings after her own workday is complete. The intern explains to you that while Mr. J has been through "a lot" in this hospital course, she feels that he needs to "just toughen up."

You wonder if the intern's dismissive reaction to Mr. J is attributable to the demanding surgical culture that has resulted in her own need to "toughen up" or perhaps other factors in her life that are influencing her. You, too, notice a similar irritation at Mr. J's seemingly cavalier suicidal statements, made in the context of what appear to be mundane and necessary tasks of his medical care. You notice a desire to take seriously Mr. J's expressions of suffering while also feeling annoyed because Mr. J's statements do not, in fact, sound "serious." In addition, you now have the burden of an additional consult to see during the day. You take note of the countertransference you're experiencing, keeping in mind that it may be informative in your approach to treating Mr. J.

When you enter Mr. J's room, you're surprised to see a burly, athletic man sitting in bed, watching reruns of an old television show. His muscular, tattooed arms provide a stark contrast to the man described in the chart who's endured a long and complicated hospital admission. You inquire about his mood, and Mr. J describes to you feeling "terminally bored," as he continues to channel surf during your interview. You remark upon the fact that he's been on the surgical unit for several weeks now and ask how he has been coping. Mr. J is dismissive when you ask him about his suicidal statements and says "listen, I got a lot of bigger problems now than wanting to kill myself." You ask what he means by this, and Mr. J replies with an exasperated tone, assuring you that he's "not gonna do anything." He rolls his eyes and replies "yes!" when you ask him if he made the suicidal statements out of frustration. As your rapport at this point is—at best—tenuous, you ask if you may speak to Mr. J's wife. He begrudgingly gives his permission. As the only time Mrs. J can visit the unit is in the evenings, you plan to go later that day to speak to her.

That evening Mrs. J arrives with their two young children in tow and appears frazzled. Mrs. J is surprised to learn that the team has requested that a psychiatrist evaluate her husband but confides that she's glad you are there. While Mr. J sits in his room with his two children in the company of the one-to-one sitter, in the hallway Mrs. J details for you the struggles her family's endured as a result of her husband being hospitalized for such a long time. With Mr. J self-employed as an independent contractor, their income has now sharply declined since he's been unable to work, which has only added to the burden of Mrs. J caring for their two children alone while working full-time. She describes to you how Mr. J has really been struggling in the hospital—he has been irritable with her, snaps at their two children, and when he thinks Mrs. J has left the hospital for the night, she has witnessed him crying in his room. To her knowledge she denies any concern that Mr. J would harm himself given his devotion to their family. He has not been drinking or using substances. You thank Mrs. J for her time, and consider your next steps, feeling more empathic toward Mr. J and his family's struggles.

The next day, Mr. J appears somewhat more amenable to speaking with you, and the tension in your interaction has been noticeably diffused. You suspect Mrs. J may have played a role in encouraging him to speak to you. You are able to complete a more thorough safety assessment on Mr. J and find that he is a low risk for suicide. Mr. J details that he voiced suicidality as a means of expressing his frustration that has been building, and with his wife unable to be present for the team's morning meetings and rounds, he feels as if shouldering this burden of discharge planning has limited his ability to cope. You suspect that Mr. J's feeling unequipped to manage this burden is a source of shame and anger for him. You can now better understand your—and the team's—reactions of dismissiveness and irritation with Mr. J as being a complementary countertransference, one in which you are experiencing the same dismissiveness with which Mr. J treats his own "weak self." Mr. J harbors toward *himself* an attitude of needing to "toughen up." With Mr. J, you validate his feelings of frustration, acknowledging to him that these feelings of powerlessness are likely not ones Mr. J often encounters in his roles as worker, husband, and father. You discuss with him the potential avenues for including his wife in his care with the team, helping to smooth his transition, engaging other members of his support system, and even addressing with social work his financial concerns about his hospitalization.

You return to the team and update them as to your conversations with Mr. J and his wife. The team had been unaware of Mr. J's wish to have his wife more included in his care and discharge planning and had been equally unaware of his financial burdens. While you offer the team a referral for Mr. J to a local cognitive-behavioral psychotherapy clinic so that he may strengthen his coping skills, you feel that your more salient recommendation lies in having paved the way toward an improved communication between him and his medical team. It is in this way that, by drawing upon your psychodynamic understanding of a patient and utilizing your countertransference, you can help the medical team navigate their patient's often uncomfortable, rageful, and frightening behaviors.

Appendix: Summary Table

	Problems	Strategies
• Patient symptoms and behaviors	• Safety: Suicidal behaviors or self-injury in hospital	• Implement a one-to-one sitter at all times with the patient, potentially also with a hospital security officer present, to ensure the patient's safety • To the best extent possible given the patient's medical needs, remove items from a patient's bedside that he or she may use to self-injure (i.e., medications from home, razors, scissors, etc.), especially if the patient has already self-harmed or voiced intent to do so in the hospital. This may require a room sweep by nursing to remove items if a patient is not forthcoming • Use the C-SSRS to assess a patient's risk level, and recommend an appropriate disposition plan to the primary team
• Provider-patient dynamics	• Provider has feelings of having "failed" the patient or being ineffective in managing the case. May mobilize in the provider a defensive sense of guilt, hopelessness, and anger at the patient thwarting his or her medical care • Via defenses of projective identification, devaluing, and acting out, the patient may engender in the provider a sense of anger and frustration	• Validate and empathize with the team's reactions. Use the understanding you've gained of the patient's emotions, motivations, and choices to help the team to find empathy for the patient • This, in turn, can help providers respond appropriately and not in a counter-therapeutic or retaliatory way • Outline active interventions to assist the team in managing difficult interactions with a patient, i.e., transparency with care plans and setting clear boundaries with patients over behaviors allowed in hospital

(continued)

	Problems	Strategies
• Inter-provider and provider-family dynamics	• Contention between different team members may indicate that a patient has used defensive splitting • The team feels nervous as to whether the patient will harm himself or herself while under their care and look to psychiatry for reassurance • The family may be surprised, alarmed, or relieved that psychiatry has been consulted for suicidality	• Provide psychoeducation to the team about this phenomena, and encourage team rounding to minimize the splitting • Educate the team about safety measures to be taken and provide clear disposition planning • Provide support to family, as well as clear guidelines for the patient's follow-up
• Patient-provider barriers	• The medical or surgical team has a limited amount of resources and time to devote to exploring the patient's psychological conflicts	• This is where your liaison role comes into play! Help the team to understand some of the patient's behaviors and reactions. This can serve to demystify the "psych" issues at hand and give the team an improved sense of agency in their care
• Hospital system barriers	• Teams may be pressured by hospital administration due to staffing limitations to limit the use of one-to-one sitters and security presence and may request that psychiatry lessen observation requirements	• Carefully evaluate a patient's suicide risk and underscore to the team to not compromise the patient's safety. Work with the team and the administration to ensure the patient requires the proper level of observation

References

1. Posner K, Brown GK, Stanley B, Brent DA, Yershova KV, Oquendo MA, Currier GW, Melvin GA, Greenhill L, Shen S, Mann JJ. The columbia–suicide severity rating scale: initial validity and internal consistency findings from three multisite studies with adolescents and adults. Am J Psychiatry. 2011;168:1266–77. https://doi.org/10.1176/appi.ajp.2011.10111704.
2. McWilliams N. Primary defensive process. In: McWilliams N, editor. Psychoanalytic diagnosis: understanding personality structure in clinical process, vol. 2. New York: Guilford Press; 2011.

Behaviors Interfering with Care

11

Anna M. Kim and Carrie Ernst

Your pager reads: "We've tried everything for Mr. M and nothing is helping—can psychiatry assess him?"

This page is both a reaction, expressed as a plea for help, and a general request for psychiatry's involvement in Mr. M's care. It is important to understand each of the two statements in this page individually as well as together. On the surface, this is a straightforward request: a psychiatric assessment. More precisely, however, the request conveys a wish for psychiatry to manage Mr. M's symptoms and behaviors. The team's expression of helplessness in the first half of the page may lead you to wonder: What behaviors is Mr. M exhibiting? How are they affecting the medical team emotionally? Are they affecting the primary team and hospital system's ability to engage in treatment planning? Mr. M may be exhibiting a range of potentially challenging behaviors, and obtaining a narrative of these can help clarify the specifics.

A. M. Kim (✉)
Icahn School of Medicine at Mount Sinai, New York, NY, USA
e-mail: akim19@northwell.edu

C. Ernst
Department of Psychiatry, Icahn School of Medicine at Mount Sinai, New York, NY, USA

Department of Medical Education, Icahn School of Medicine at Mount Sinai, New York, NY, USA
e-mail: Carrie.ernst@mssm.edu

A. Gorun et al. (eds.), *The Psychiatric Consult*,
https://doi.org/10.1007/978-3-031-26837-3_11

Perhaps he is verbally and physically disruptive, threatening to harm others or himself, struggling with communication, demanding frequent interaction, or quietly refusing treatment. Understanding what created the team's feeling of helplessness that prompted a psychiatric consult will guide you to be the most helpful to the primary team. Note that the team's reaction is to move to action—a psychiatric consult to assess the patient. What is the team expecting from the consultation? And is it realistic? Your first step is to find out more about these challenges by speaking to the team before seeing Mr. M.

Clinical Scenario

You take a look at the chart and discover that Mr. M is 65 years old and has a history of cigarette use and chronic obstructive lung disease. He was hospitalized for severe pneumonia and recommended to stay in the hospital for treatment including intravenous (IV) antibiotics. There is not much information regarding his psychosocial history. The chart is inundated with nursing and medical notes documenting that Mr. M is "uncooperative" and "refusing care."

You call the medical resident to obtain more information. What does she think is happening? Why the call now? The medical resident explains that she is exasperated. She has explained to Mr. M numerous times what treatment he will need to get better. However, he does not seem to listen or register the information. She is concerned that he will get worse and that a worsening infection without treatment could result in sepsis and death. She also feels angry because she feels she has done everything she can to try to help. Her feeling of helplessness has been increasing, and she is calling you now as she does not know what more there is "to do" for Mr. M if he is refusing the antibiotics that would treat his pneumonia. She is not sure what is happening to Mr. M or if he has any psychiatric history and asks for your help.

Scenario 1: Psychological Factors Affecting Another Medical Condition

You continue your discussion with the medical resident who adds that Mr. M has also made vague suicidal statements to a staff member taking care of him last night, and they added a one to one to observe him. The nurse said that he made the statement after she had been busy with a medical emergency with another patient and was not able to respond immediately to his request for a medication to help with his shortness of breath. He said that "maybe I should kill myself so I can get someone in here to pay attention to me." He has also made insulting and derogatory statements towards various doctors and nurses which has caused them considerable distress. They have expressed during rounds that they try to avoid interacting with him because of this. The resident has noticed, however, that there is one nurse whom he has asked to be assigned to him for multiple nights and who will defend him on rounds when others complain about him. This particular nurse has caused considerable conflict as she will page the doctors continuously asking for more medications to treat his shortness of breath and thinks that the team is not treating him fairly. You ask her what the nurse says, and the medical resident tells you that the nurse says she has "time to listen and understand him" and that he has expressed being "afraid and left alone to die" to her. You think to yourself that this help seeking expression contradicts the overnight suicidal statements and you will include that in your risk assessment when you evaluate him.

You ask how Mr. M is doing medically. She informs you that he has been short of breath since admission and that, despite their recommendation that antibiotics would help cure his underlying symptoms, he has not agreed to this treatment. Instead, he has asked for multiple medications to treat his shortness of breath symptomatically. She says that, as expected, these medications do not fully treat his symptoms without the antibiotics. He becomes frustrated that he is still short of breath and asks for an alternative medication because the current one is ineffective, and then the new medication ultimately also fails. As the resident, she is constantly getting paged by his nurse about his shortness of breath bothering him. She tells you that he has an elevated white blood cell count, that his chest X-ray demonstrates an opacity in the right lower lobe, and that he has been febrile, but otherwise his vitals have been stable and other laboratory tests have been unremarkable. His urine drug screen did come back positive for cannabis and she wonders out loud to you if that could be the cause of his challenging behavior.

The information you see in the chart confirms what the medical resident has said. Under the medication administration section, multiple medications for dyspnea and anxiety have been ordered, stopped, and restarted. You start to think of a differential prior to seeing the patient based on what you have learned so far, including potentially inflexible personality traits resulting in general poor coping in the hospital setting such as in psychological factors affecting other medical conditions [1]. You also want to make sure to consider the contribution of substances, medications, and medical conditions to his anxiety and behavioral dysregulation.

Following a discussion with the team, a review of the chart, and a possible differential, you now have a better understanding of the challenging day-to-day interactions with Mr. M. Mr. M seems to be engaging in help-seeking and help-rejecting behaviors [2–4] with the team, as evidenced by his repeatedly asking for help but then refusing the treatment that would help him. His hostility has caused the team significant distress that results in them wanting to avoid him, while at the same time he appears to try to engage with the team incessantly for medications to treat his symptoms. When staff did not respond to his request for a medication, he replied with a threatening suicidal statement. You also suspect Mr. M has been "splitting" [2–4] the team members, that is, seeing each member of the team reactively as absolutely "good" or "bad." Such rigid division by the patient often manifests as a form of coping and can result in a lack of collaborative functioning within a team. You ask that the resident, the head nurse, and his nurse for the day (who happens to be the nurse that he has requested multiple times) to join your interview in an effort to reduce the split that the patient has generated.

Upon entering the room, you notice that Mr. M is crying and appears dysphoric. You introduce yourself and the other team members and the reason you were asked to speak to him, including that he declined the primary team's recommendation for antibiotics. He immediately starts listing a number of complaints, including that the nurses do not understand him, that the doctors only want to treat him in order to "kick [him] out," and that the hospital system is ill equipped to "respond to their own sick patients in distress" noting "the call button isn't even working… or maybe the nurses just don't care enough to respond to it!" He is now no longer tearful but is shouting and angry. He tells you the hospital does not care if he dies and that the team will understand his suffering once he cuts his arms and bleeds to death. You attempt to verbally de-escalate him by rephrasing and reflecting back his statements [2], but do not directly challenge them. You also attempt to remain calm despite his hostility, which eventually results in him becoming calmer as well. Mr. M starts to talk about other things that are making him upset, including that his family has not visited him during this hospitalization. He feels "rejected by everyone…except for that one nurse…she's the only reason I'm still here, still alive." The nurse smiles and responds positively to Mr. M's comment. She is on the "good" side of the split. The head nurse turns away. The medical resident is expressionless, but checks her pager repeatedly, appearing to be losing patience. You are witnessing the dynamics that are at play between the team members in the room as he is speaking.

You think it might be helpful to put into words the dynamics in the room and what you hypothesize Mr. M may be experiencing. You point out to Mr. M that he seems to want help while at the same time rejecting it as well, and then you ask him his thoughts on this. He tells you that he does want help, but the team is unable to help him adequately. You ask Mr. M what adequate help would look like, and he explains "people who actually care." You reflect to yourself that he has created a dynamic where his medical team is unable to help him in the way he wants and wonder whether this has also happened with his family who has not visited him. You decide to ask him if you can call his family to see if they may be able to help in understanding Mr. M and also potentially ally with you in having Mr. M take the antibiotics he needs. You ask him if you can call his family, and Mr. M appears to brighten and say "yeah, you can call my girlfriend, and be sure to tell her that if she doesn't come it'll be the last time she can see me before I'm dead." The pattern of reacting with hostility and suicidal statements when the patient is feeling he is not getting enough attention appears clearer to you. When you ask him whether he expresses frustration towards others about not feeling he is getting what he needs by threatening suicide, he agrees with this and says he will not actually do it, but he knows that saying he will kill himself usually gets people to "actually do something." You ask him if he has ever acted on wanting to kill himself, which he denies, and he adds that he has been "using that trick for years."

You quickly screen for major mood, anxiety, and psychotic symptoms which he denies. His cognitive functioning is normal. He denies any substance use except for episodic marijuana "to mellow me out." He denies any psychiatric hospitalizations, and there is no family history of mental illness. At this point, the patient does not meet criteria for any mood, anxiety, or psychotic disorder, and you are conceptualizing him as a man who expresses his distress and needs via suicidal statements and hostility. You ask him whether he plans on hurting himself while in the hospital, which he says to "only if it'll get someone to pay attention to me around here." You decide to continue the order for a sitter to observe him while you get more information but are less concerned that he represents an acute suicidal risk given the chronic nature of his statements and that he has never acted on them.

When you call the phone number he gave you, you are surprised to hear that the woman who picks up broke up with him 3 months ago and she is his ex-girlfriend. She tells you that Mr. M smokes marijuana "in excess," especially when upset. She reports that Mr. M does not have a history of self-injury or actually making a suicide attempt, but has threatened to cut himself or kill himself in the past multiples times. She does not know of any outpatient psychiatrist but is aware of many emergency room visits after he was feeling upset about some aspect of his medical care and saying he was suicidal. She has received multiple calls from these emergency room providers, and they have discharged him after speaking to her. You explain his current medical condition and how he is declining the antibiotics that were offered to him. She sighs and says "I'll call him – he does this all the time to get my attention."

At this point, you have a better understanding of Mr. M's patterns of coping and acting on statements of distress. Although one could make the case for diagnosing Mr. M with a personality disorder during this hospitalization, you decide to hold off considering the current acute medical stressors of his hospitalization. Soon after speaking to his ex-girlfriend, you receive a page from the resident that Mr. M is now agreeing to take the antibiotics. Now that he has agreed to treatment, your role at this point is to help the primary team assess his safety and help them contain Mr. M's displays of distress and affective lability without disengaging from him.

In this scenario, the staff and residents of the medical team are struggling to manage this behaviorally challenging patient. Clarifying Mr. M's contradictory behavior and tendency to "act out" when feeling overwhelmed rather than expressing his needs helps the patient assume responsibility rather than externalize onto the team that they are not being helpful or do not care. Recognizing this for both the patient and team can help them understand the dynamics that impact their ability to treat this patient.

Scenario 2: Cultural and Communication Barriers

According to the resident during your initial phone call, Mr. M has been refusing IV antibiotics for his pneumonia for several days. She is confused as to why he does not want to take it—she thought maybe it has something to do with using an IV, but taking the antibiotic in an oral form would not adequately treat his infection. The resident tells you that their service has been busy, and because of that, she has not had the time to gather too much information about his social background, but knows that he recently immigrated from China to be near his family. She attempted to ask him about the antibiotics and why he does not want to take them, and he just shakes his head "no." When she then asks him to explain why he is saying no, he shakes his head "no" again. The medical resident tried to use the interpreter services since English is his second language, but he continued to shake his head "no" even when using his native language of Cantonese. You ask the medical resident about behaviors indicative of delirium or clear concerns regarding safety of Mr. M which she denied. She says he is always alert and answers her orientation questions accurately and has not been confused.

You decide to review the chart for further clues. The vitals are notable for tachycardia, fever, and a decreased pulse oxygen. Laboratory tests demonstrate an elevated white blood cell count. Chest X-ray reveals an opacity in the lower lobe of the right lung. You next review the clinical notes and medications. There you observe that an interpreter service has been used and recorded in some of the interdisciplinary notes. Other notes document Mr. M's "refusal of care," but do not elaborate on the details of this. There is a paucity of documentation about who the patient is, but you do see that a daughter is listed as an emergency contact.

Upon entering the room, you first note that Mr. M is sitting calmly in a chair looking out the window. You ask Mr. M his preferred language and he replies "Cantonese," and you get an interpreter on the phone. When you ask him what brought him to the hospital, he tells you that he has a "small cough, but it will go away." Mr. M notes that his daughter visited him at home, and when she noticed him coughing, she insisted on driving him to the hospital. He elaborates that the doctors have told him that he has a lung infection and that he needs IV antibiotics. However, he does not completely agree. He feels well and plans on managing the symptoms "naturally." Mr. M tells you that he almost never seeks medical care and that he does not understand why he is meeting with a psychiatrist. He informs you that he is not "crazy" and prefers using the herbal supplements he has at home. Mr. M is additionally concerned that the costs of being in the hospital will be exorbitant and a burden both to him and his daughter.

You notice how easily he engaged in a conversation with you, which was not what you were expecting based on the resident's report. You start to wonder about cultural factors [5, 6] that may be contributing to some of the interactions with Mr. M. What else does he prefer about the "natural" supplement aside from cost? What does he make of his daughter's concern? You start to ask questions aimed at understanding his views about medical care. His mother died of lung cancer in an American hospital after a prolonged, complicated, and painful treatment course. Mr. M becomes tearful while describing this experience and tells you that he does not want to succumb to a similar experience. You reflect to yourself that perhaps his current experience in the hospital is reminiscent of these past, negative memories of the healthcare system. You explain to Mr. M that a psychiatrist is asked to see a patient when there are differences between the patient and doctors regarding what kind of treatment is best and not because someone is "crazy." You ask about his sleep, anxiety, and mood symptoms and assess for the presence of psychotic symptoms. You also ask about thoughts of wanting to end his life or hurt others. His psychiatric review of systems is unremarkable.

Mr. M's narrative describes how distrust of the medical system due to his family's experience, as well as communication and cultural factors [7, 8], can impact treatment. Mr. M is not "difficult" in the sense that he has been agitated, overtly hostile, provocative, or manipulative. Rather, he has been declining care due to a lack of trust and prior aversive experiences and losses related to the medical system. There is also a lack of understanding of his medical condition as well as why IV antibiotics are indicated, indicating an impairment in communication between Mr. M and primary team. Your role as a consultation-liaison psychiatrist is to facilitate communication in an effort to bridge the two, while ultimately ensuring Mr. M's preferences are attended to.

Mr. M reiterates that he is "fine". You remember he has a daughter and think to yourself that not only will talking to her help you understand Mr. M better, but that her support may be critical for her father's engagement in treatment. Mr. M provides consent for you speak with his daughter and agrees that it would be helpful to involve her in his care since she is the one who wanted him to come to the hospital.

Mr. M's daughter explains that she has been unaware that he has been refusing to take antibiotics. She states she brought her father to the hospital for worsening cough, difficulty breathing, and fever. Her father generally does not like physicians and that his mistrust and avoidance of Western medicine has been a long-standing belief. He prefers acupuncture, exercise, and traditional herbal treatments [5, 6]. She agrees to meet with you, her father, an in-person interpreter, and the primary team to discuss a plan and to support both her father's needs and treatment decision-making.

During the meeting, you are able to use questions from the Kleinman's model of illness [7] to help you and the primary team understand Mr. M's perspective. He believes that his pneumonia was caused by the cold weather and his own stress, in addition to believing that it could be quickly treated with "natural" treatments. He also fears that more intensive interventions will cause him harm as it did to his mother, to the extent that he may possibly die. After the meeting, you talk with the team about how cultural factors can be interpreted as Mr. M seeming uncooperative or challenging, but that his choices in his treatment stem from the whole of his life experience. Rather than approaching this as a psychiatric symptom, the use of an in-person interpreter or encouraging the presence of a trusted family member at bedside during treatment discussions can be helpful in reconciling differences between a medical team and a patient.

In addition to easing communication, as the consultation-liaison psychiatrist, you would also like to educate medical teams on existing guidelines regarding cultural sensitivity [7, 8]. National measures have encouraged hospital systems to recruit and retain staff members who reflect the cultural diversity of the population, to encourage cultural competency training of providers, and to provide patients culturally appropriate health education materials. Structured, exploratory approaches, such as Kleinman's model of illness, can help physicians understand how patients perceive their health in the broader context of life and help clinicians explore cross-cultural understandings [7]. You also encourage the use of patient-centered language and education, addressing specific patient concerns, and incorporating preferred complementary medicine treatments where safe and appropriate, in an effort to ensure that patients feel heard and supported in their care preferences. The resident decides to look up the herbal supplement Mr. M is referring to and sees that there are no potential interactions or harm to him taking it. The patient, his daughter, and the primary team agree for Mr. M to take both the herbal supplement and the antibiotics as a compromise.

In this scenario, staff and the primary medical team feel frustrated by Mr. M's lack of agreement with treatment, and they are having difficulty determining the cause. Identifying what is impacting care and providing the team with an approach for managing these challenges is key. In this case, an issue of cultural competency on the part of the team and prior negative experiences on the part of the patient contribute to a dynamic where treatment is stuck, not a psychiatric disorder. Involving sources of support whom Mr. M trusts allows you to clarify aspects of his history, life narrative, cultural perspectives, and care preferences. These are vital in facilitating rapport and communication between the team and Mr. M.

Scenario 3: Delirium

After returning the consult page and speaking with the medical resident, you ask more specific questions concerning Mr. M's recent behavior: What has he been doing to "refuse" care? Is this the first time or has it occurred on multiple occasions? The resident informs you that Mr. M has been irritable and restless, pacing in his room, shouting when no one is around, and making inappropriate comments to staff. The resident elaborates that she suspects he's "antisocial" and is using racial slurs that are upsetting to the other patient in the room, though she also notes he has seemed confused and they needed restraints to stop him from pulling out his IV. She thinks he might be a bit delirious, but that he clearly also has a personality disorder given how intentionally he seems to insult staff. You think to yourself that antisocial personality disorder is defined as a pervasive pattern of disregard for and violation of the rights of others indicated by recklessness, irresponsibility, and a lack of remorse since early adulthood [1]. The resident is unaware of Mr. M's baseline functioning prior to hospitalization or psychiatric history. The team emphasizes that they called you because he is refusing antibiotics but also because they need help managing his aggressive behaviors.

You begin to review the chart, starting with the vitals. You note that Mr. M is hypoxic, tachypneic, and tachycardic. You next look at his laboratory tests, which are remarkable for an elevated white blood cell count and lactate. Liver and thyroid functioning appears normal. His kidney function was initially impaired, but appears to have normalized with IV fluids. Urine drug screen was negative on admission. Imaging reveals opacities on Mr. M's chest x-ray indicative of pneumonia. His electrocardiogram is unremarkable. He has not received any psychiatric medications preemptively from the primary team. You continue to review the rest of his medications, vigilant to select antibiotics, opioids, benzodiazepines, corticosteroids, and drugs with anticholinergic and antihistaminergic properties that can worsen delirium, which is high on your differential diagnosis, given his abnormal vitals, medical illness, and agitation [9, 10]. Following a review of the vitals, labs, imaging, and medications, you begin a more in-depth chart review and uncover a cognitive exam completed several months ago. You see that he scored a 24/30 on the Montreal Cognitive Assessment (MoCA) [11]. You think about how patients with a history of mild neurocognitive deficits can be more predisposed to delirium.

You continue your in-depth chart review to look for any psychiatric history and to locate any available notes that may hint at his baseline, including personality traits alluded to in prior medical documentation and by the resident. He appears to see his primary care doctor in a clinic for the past 10 years, and there is no documentation regarding any formal psychiatric history, including depressive, manic, or psychotic episodes, and no noted history of anxiety symptoms. You learn that Mr. M has had sustained employment in real estate and is married with two sons. This information suggests against personality disorder, where life-long, inflexible patterns of adapting interfere with multiple facets of a person's life [1]. He was in a car accident 7 years ago and suffered a mild traumatic brain injury (TBI). Head injury additionally could predispose him to delirium. His family had subsequently reported a change in his personality—he had become more impatient, impulsive, and disinhibited. The chart does not indicate any history of seizures following his TBI, and the lack of anti-epileptics in his medication history confirms this information. Mr. M does not have any other history psychiatric illness and has never been in outpatient psychiatric care. There is no history of self-harm, suicide, or violence. Mr. M smokes cigarettes and does not have a documented history of alcohol or illicit substance use. There is no family history of mental illness. There is no history of emotion, physical, or sexual trauma or history of legal problems.

You find that the chart review was very informative given the low likelihood of obtaining reliable information from Mr. M in his current state. You quickly review a possible differential prior to seeing him. You are considering a neurocognitive disorder, delirium, substance intoxication or withdrawal, a major psychiatric illness such as bipolar disorder or a psychotic disorder, or perhaps a personality disorder—although this is much lower on your differential.

As you enter the medical unit, you can hear Mr. M shouting, disrupting the milieu, and drawing considerable staff attention to his room. The primary team had placed Mr. M on one-to-one observation, and the sitter is making efforts to calm and reassure him. You note that Mr. M is laying in bed with soft mitten restraints on his hands. You ask the sitter for their direct observations of Mr. M's behavior: prior to the 2-point restraint, he again was trying to pull out his IV, grabbing and throwing objects at staff, and scratching his face as well as staff members who approached him.

You ask Mr. M directly, "You seem upset about something, what's going on?" He says he does not understand why he is "locked up" and wants to go home. You ask him where he is and he is able to name the hospital but identifies the year as 1974 and cannot tell you the correct month. You assess his attention by asking him to spell the word "world" backwards—he quickly loses track and perseverates on "D-L." It becomes clear that additional interview may not be productive and collateral information is important for understanding Mr. M's presentation.

You call Mr. M's wife who is his emergency contact, and she confirms that he is usually a polite, and intelligent man. The TBI changed his personality a little but he has never had problems functioning interpersonally or at work. She tells you he appeared more confused and had behavioral changes about a day prior to his hospitalization. She indicates that at some visits she makes to the hospital, he does seem more like his typical self. You think to yourself that this means he has a fluctuating mental status. You are increasingly confident in your diagnosis of hyperactive delirium, given the acute onset and waxing and waning symptoms, the alterations in orientation and attention, and the cognitive deficits [9, 10].

You speak to the team about the objective mental status exam findings and symptoms you have observed and elicited from the patient and clarify to them that he is not "refusing care" but is delirious. You make recommendations to initiate a neuroleptic given his degree of agitation and its interference with his medical care and safety. You outline precautions for reducing the incidence and prolongation of delirium. Importantly, you explain to the medical resident that not every "difficult" patient has a personality disorder diagnosis and that behaviors that can appear volitional may in fact be part of an underlying medical diagnosis. You elaborate that the history you obtained from the wife does not indicate a lifelong pattern of recklessness, irresponsibility, or disregard for others as in antisocial personality disorder [1]. You identify Mr. M's agitated and aggressive behavior as related to delirium as opposed to pathological character traits. Even in the absence of delirium, hospitalization may lead patients to act in uncharacteristically challenging ways that would not meet criteria for a personality disorder.

You add to your differential diagnosis an underlying neurocognitive disorder due to TBI, and note that this may complicate and increase his risk of delirium. This diagnosis is suggested by Mr. M's MoCA score, taking into account his education level and baseline functioning. You consider Mr. M's longer-term management and recommend that the team refer Mr. M for neuropsychological testing following hospitalization and once his delirium clears for further diagnostic workup.

This case is not unique. It is not uncommon for primary teams to misattribute unpleasant or aggressive behavior to a psychiatric disorder. One aspect of your role as the consulting psychiatrist is to take a step back and help teams understand their own feelings, reactions, and associated stigma. In differentiating a personality disorder from other diagnoses in the hospital setting, additional information from collateral is key. Collateral information and a full chart review provide a longitudinal perspective and assist in identifying stable personality traits versus patterned behavioral and interpersonal difficulties, or acute deviations from baseline that may be unique to setting or circumstances. Dismissive, hostile, and inflexible characteristics in patients can evoke feelings of frustration, defeat, or anger. This could potentially lead providers to make a premature diagnostic assumption of a "personality disorder" rather than appreciating contextual variability, the role of medical comorbidities, and psychological responses to illness. In these cases, the consultation-liaison psychiatrist can contextualize the patient's symptoms in an effort to support provider compassion and empathy.

Appendix: Summary Table [1–11]

	Problems	Strategies
• Patient symptoms and behaviors	• Maladaptive personality traits (e.g., hopelessness, acting out) • Lack of trust in the healthcare system • Poor health literacy • Neurocognitive disorder • Functional impairment	• Contain distress • Limit set • Avoid splitting • Build a therapeutic alliance • Provide clarification and context to concerns • Encourage approach that involves family and friends • Educate the team that unpleasant personalities or behavioral disturbances can have causes that are not psychiatric • Provide cultural understanding
• Provider-patient dynamics	• Provider feeling frustrated • Provider feeling helpless • Patient acting out • Provider avoidance or disengagement • Provider defensiveness • Patient feeling hopeless	• Validate provider and patient emotions • Help the team develop compassion and model empathy • Help the primary team understand ongoing dynamics and enactments between provider and patient—More specifically that behaviors from both sides reinforce unwanted outcome
• Patient-provider barriers	• Dynamics can act as barriers to treatment • Lack of appropriate translator services • Lack of culturally competent information	• Emphasize curiosity, respect, and a nonjudgmental approach • Address concerns in a specific, concrete manner
• Hospital system barriers	• Insidious creation of a culture of discrimination • Negative countertransference becomes the new hospital "standard" reaction to certain patients • Superficial engagement leading to readmissions	• Programs for cultural competency and humility with concrete pathways to facilitate patient care • Encourage discussion of dynamics between patient and provider and hospital • Foster and reward collaboration • Address causes of readmissions

References

1. Desk reference to the diagnostic criteria from DSM-5 (R). Arlington, VA: The American Psychiatric Association Publishing; 2013.
2. Shea SC. Psychiatric interviewing: the art of understanding: a practical guide for psychiatrists, psychologists, counselors, social workers, nurses, and other mental health professionals. 2nd ed. Philadelphia, PA: Saunders; 1998.
3. Groves JE. Taking care of the hateful patient. N Engl J Med. 1978;298:883–7.
4. Gunderson JG, Links P (Collaborator). Handbook of good psychiatric management for borderline personality disorder. Washington, DC: The American Psychiatric Association Publishing; 2014.
5. Chung VCH, et al. Views on traditional Chinese medicine amongst Chinese population: a systematic review of qualitative and quantitative studies. Health Expect. 2014;17(5):622–36.
6. Xu Q, et al. The quest for modernisation of traditional Chinese medicine. BMC Complement Altern Med. 2013;13:132.
7. Centers for Disease Control and Prevention. Practical strategies for culturally competent evaluation. Atlanta: US Department of Health and Human Services; 2014. https://www.cdc.gov/asthma/program_eval/cultural_competence_guide.pdf.
8. Office of Minority Health, US Department of Health and Human Services. Cultural and linguistic competency. https://minorityhealth.hhs.gov/cultural-and-linguistic-competency.
9. Leentjens AFG, Meagher DJ. Delirium. In: Levenson J, editor. The American Psychiatric Association Publishing textbook of psychosomatic medicine and consult liaison psychiatry. 3rd ed. Washingon, DC: The American Psychiatric Association Publishing; 2019.
10. Caplan JP. Delirious patients. In: Stern TA, Freudenreich O, Smith FA, Fricchione GL, Rosenbaum JF, editors. Massachusetts General Hospital handbook of general hospital psychiatry. 7th ed. Amsterdam: Elsevier; 2018.
11. Nasreddine ZS, et al. The Montreal Cognitive Assessment, MoCA: a brief screening tool for mild cognitive impairment. J Am Geriatr Soc. 2005;53(4):195–9.

Further Reading

American Psychiatric Association. Best practice highlights for treating diverse patient populations. https://www.psychiatry.org/psychiatrists/diversity/education/bestpractice-highlights.

Goldberg JF, Ernst CL. Managing the side effects of psychotropic medications. 2nd ed. Washington, DC: The American Psychiatric Association Publishing; 2018.

12 Adjustment Disorder

Jasdeep Sandhu and Omar Mirza

Your pager reads: "I think the patient is depressed, can you talk to him?"

The word "depression" can have different meanings for physicians and non-physicians alike. When a provider expresses concern that a patient is "depressed," the psychiatric consultant should initially maintain a broad differential diagnosis, along with curiosity about the observations that prompted their concern. In this pager request, the medical team is not only asking the diagnostic question of whether or not this patient has a depressive disorder but may also be implying a number of other questions. An initial task for the consultant is to clarify what has led the primary team to think that the patient may be depressed. Perhaps the medical team observed that the patient is tearful and dysthymic, withdrawn and quiet, or are concerned that the patient is not participating in care productively. The patient themselves may have expressed feeling sad, been isolated, or expressed a desire for hastened death or simply wanting to "talk" to someone. Alternatively, members of the primary team may be feeling hope-

J. Sandhu (✉)
Department of Psychiatry, Dell Medical School- The University of Texas at Austin, Austin, TX, USA
e mail: jsandhu@mygbhp.com

O. Mirza
Department of Psychiatry, Harlem Hospital, New York, NY, USA

A. Gorun et al. (eds.), *The Psychiatric Consult*,
https://doi.org/10.1007/978-3-031-26837-3_12

less about their patient's medical condition and believe that the patient must similarly be feeling distressed or demoralized.

To clarify the question, you aim to first identify the phenomenology of the patient's symptoms—what signs of depression or concerning behaviors has the primary team noted? What exactly is the patient or the medical team experiencing and attributing to "depression"? These questions may also help to identify a process-related problem, such as a patient declining treatment recommendations, or demanding more time than the team feels they have to offer. Additional questions may help to add important context to the patient's presentation—does the patient have a psychiatric history? Has there been a change in the patient's demeanor, and have the concerning symptoms and behaviors evolved over the course of their hospitalization? How does the patient engage interpersonally and in treatment at their baseline?

Patient safety is of utmost importance when accepting a consultation, particularly when the primary medical team identifies the presence of agitation or aggression, hyperactive delirium, psychosis, or acute distress and depressive changes that raise concern for suicidal ideation. When consulted for depression, it is pertinent to ask the primary team about suicidal ideation, plans, or behaviors expressed by the patient or observed by team members and to assess the acuity of the consultation. If safety concerns are present, it may be prudent to instruct the team to initiate a higher level of observation (e.g., one-to-one observation status) to ensure the immediate safety of the provider and patient before further assessment can take place.

Clinical Scenario

You return the pager request and speak to the oncology fellow who requested the consultation. The consult is for Mr. Q, a 55-year-old man who was recently diagnosed with non-small cell lung cancer and is now postoperative day 4 from complete surgical resection of the primary tumor. The oncology team reports that the surgery was completed without complications and that the patient is going to start treatment with chemotherapy while in the hospital. The team notes that the patient has seemed "down" and withdrawn and had reported feeling anxious and uncertain about his treatment, despite receiving positive news about the surgical outcome and medical therapy options.

The primary medical team feels optimistic about Mr. Q's prognosis and had hoped that his apparent anxiety and low mood would improve once he completed his surgery. On rounds this morning, the patient told the fellow that he feels he is persistently worried and "unable to find relief." The team asked him if he felt depressed, and Mr. Q endorsed feeling sad and overwhelmed. The primary team did not ask follow-up questions to better understand the nature of Mr. Q's distress. The fellow explains that Mr. Q has "seemed different" since his surgery and has been difficult to motivate and engage throughout the subsequent treatment process. The fellow had also been involved in Mr. Q's care in the oncology clinic prior to this planned hospital admission and notes that Mr. Q had expressed ambivalence about treatment since receiving the diagnosis and required multiple meetings before opting to move forward with surgery and chemotherapy at the urging of his spouse and oncologist.

You ask questions to begin to assess if Mr. Q has exhibited behavioral issues or signs of delirium over the course of his hospitalization. The fellow denies both and states that until recently he has been accepting of ongoing care and participating in treatment planning and care. The fellow confirms that the patient seems to have supportive family available and that his wife visits frequently and has been very involved in his day-to-day care in the hospital. She has similarly expressed concern to the medical team that Mr. Q has seemed increasingly depressed. The fellow requests your recommendations for treatment of depression and anxiety and adds that "The patient really needs someone to talk to about everything he has been going through."

Scenario 1: Demoralization

As you continue speaking with the oncology fellow, you wonder if the team is struggling with their own feelings of hopelessness and frustration in treating Mr. Q. The medical team is concerned that the patient continues to appear withdrawn and dysphoric despite their hope for improvement over time and with active medical interventions. The fellow notes that Mr. Q had also mentioned on rounds that he was feeling uncertain about continuing with his treatment, and the medical team would like for you to assess for an underlying psychiatric contribution to his presentation. You begin to hypothesize that the fellow my be trying to distance himself from uncomfortable thoughts of self-reproach, or feelings of failure for the inability to "fix" the patient's ongoing distress with medical interventions, in addition to the stated concern about his declining treatment engagement. By requesting assistance from another specialist, he can mitigate some of the feelings of frustration and powerlessness, while making proactive interventions and ensuring the patient is being cared for psychologically and medically.

You review the chart to gather history and in the process begin to develop a preliminary differential diagnosis. You find no documented psychiatric history and no psychotropic medications that might indicate a preexisting mood disorder. You review his vital signs for hypertension and tachycardia—which could serve as broad indicators of other factors impacting Mr. Q's behavior, such as substance use or withdrawal, pain, anxiety, or agitation—and his vital signs are stable and within normal range. Nursing notes comment on Mr. Q being calm and cooperative, and there is no documented evidence of disruptive, agitated, or aggressive behaviors, which is consistent with the team's observations. Finally, you review Mr. Q's recent labs and find abnormalities in his complete blood count which developed postoperatively. You note that the patient had a microcytic anemia at the time of his admission and experienced a further drop in hemoglobin after surgery, symptoms of which—including fatigue, malaise, and concentration difficulties—can contribute to Mr. Q struggling during his recovery from surgery and appearing to the team to be depressed. You review the medication administration record in Mr. Q's chart and find that he is on standing opioid analgesics, which are being rapidly tapered. Opioids can contribute to sedation, impact mood, and increase risk for delirium. Conversely, inadequately managed pain may manifest in agitation, impact participation in care, and contribute to challenging behaviors and interpersonal dynamics between the patient, primary team, and nursing staff. You make note to assess Mr. Q for delirium, constipation, somnolence, and pain as part of your evaluation, as each may play a role in his concerning clinical presentation.

You meet with Mr. Q, and introduce your role on the treatment team, and observe that he appears reactive, engaged, and with greater affective range than you had anticipated based on the fellow's description. Mr. Q reviews his history and goes on to describe his initial sense of "shock" after being informed he has cancer, followed by feelings of despair about his diagnoses and uncertainty about his future. Mr. Q reports struggling more after surgery, as he feels weak and has been depending on nurses to get out of bed, bathe, and transfer to the commode. You note the patient is describing feeling uncomfortable in the sick role and that he sounds more disheartened and helpless rather than overtly melancholic as you prompt him about his symptoms and experience in the hospital. Mr. Q elaborates on a sense of profound frustration from the impact of his illness on his functioning, noting a prolonged period of fatigue, weight loss, and shortness of breath prior to his diagnosis, and now being dependent on medical staff and feeling uncertain of if he will ever recover. You ask him about his life and functioning before he became sick, and he highlights his identity as a husband and father who has always been healthy and active, productive, independent, and a leader in his career field. Mr. Q follows this description with a sigh and remarks "now look at me, a feeble, sick *patient*."

As Mr. Q describes his experience of being medically ill, you recognize that he feels demoralized and identify a shift in his self-perception, including a sense of disempowerment, incompetence, and helplessness [1]. The patient's experience also seems to parallel the feelings of demoralization that the primary medical team may be experiencing when they interact with the patient. You question Mr. Q about any other sources of distress, and he endorses physical symptoms associated with both depression and cancer, including fatigue, a decline in appetite, and poor sleep, which have persisted since his diagnosis and have worsened during the

2-week period prior to surgery. He reports generally feeling "down" and frustrated and has been crying the last few nights. You ask about sources of support and Mr. Q says that he appreciates his wife visiting and tries to "put on a brave face for her," but has been having ruminative worries that cancer and chemotherapy will impact his functioning, which may consequently affect his wife and their relationship.

You ask about pain, given that its persistence can play a significant role in patient distress and demoralization if inadequately controlled. Mr. Q explains that the medical team was quick to respond to his initial postoperative pain with medication, but have been rapidly reducing the dose, and he has been experiencing increased pain and difficulty tolerating most physical activity. You note that it is challenging for Mr. Q to recognize or share the hopeful perspective that the primary team has been communicating about his surgical outcome, which may be a reflection of his ongoing pain and demoralization. The disconnect between Mr. Q's loss of morale and pessimistic view of his future and the primary medical team's optimism and expectation for post-surgical relief may be contributing to the primary team's concern about his mood and progress.

You share with the patient how major life changes that have an effect on a sense of well-being and identity—such as being diagnosed with a major medical condition that feels out of someone's control—can lead to feelings of sadness, hopelessness, or even anger. You encourage Mr. Q to share these feelings with his family and suggest that ongoing psychotherapy can be helpful for coping with his diagnosis and treatment and over the course of his recovery. You help him to identify strategies to actively address some of his symptoms, using the opportunity to counsel him on important behavioral interventions for sleep hygiene, exercise, and prioritizing personally meaningful activities (e.g., spending time with family and friends, participating in his hobbies and work). You also speak with his wife by telephone, who reports noticing signs and symptoms of mood changes and anxiety consistent with what the patient had described. She expresses concern that he seems to be missing "that spark he had" before his diagnosis. You share with Mr. Q's wife that her husband seems to benefit from time she spends with him in the hospital and her continued support will be critical in his recovery. By understanding his feelings and supporting his adjustment to the cancer diagnosis and recent changes in his functioning, she can help him to restore his sense of resiliency and independence, which are negatively affected when demoralized.

You find the oncology team after evaluating Mr. Q and explain your diagnostic impression of adjustment disorder with depressed mood. You educate the team about how his illness has challenged the patient's sense of self—of being independent, competent, and in good health—and the resultant depressive response he is experiencing. You discuss the concept of *demoralization* and provide the team with psychoeducation regarding how it is differentiated from depression in the case of Mr. Q. You define demoralization as distress and loss of morale as a result of a failure to cope with a major stressor, which can result in perceived feelings of powerlessness, impotence, incompetence, hopelessness, helplessness in the ability to affect the outcome of the situation, and injury to the person's self-esteem [2]. Demoralization may be present in approximately one-third of medically ill patients, regardless of the presence or absence of an underlying psychiatric disorder [1]. When demoralized, a patient might feel helpless and incompetent in their ability to cope and have an increased sense of uncertainty around which direction to take in their care as their sense of self and expectations have shifted. While dysphoria and loss of hope are often present in both major depression and demoralization, the demoralized patient typically retains the ability to experience some pleasure in hedonic activity, feels connected with and can make use of support within their relationships, retains a sense of motivation, and can recognize their distress as a reaction to an external stressor. In contrast, the presence of a depressive disorder may be identified by prominent neurovegetative depressive symptoms, anhedonia, apathy, and a sense of isolation and guilt [3]. In your assessment of Mr. Q, you are able to use these distinguishing features to rule-out the presence of major depressive disorder and identify his distress as a response to difficulties coping with his medical and functional changes.

The distinction between demoralization and a major depressive episode is important for understanding and formulating the patient's response to their medical circumstances and selecting effective treatment interventions [4]. Individual psychotherapy, engagement in support groups, and encouraging connectedness within important relationships can be helpful as Mr. Q recovers [1, 3]. Meaning-centered therapy and dignity therapy are specific psychotherapeutic modalities that can be particularly effective for the demoralized patient, as well as supportive or cognitive behavioral interventions that focus on existential distress, grief, and restoring hope, as well as identifying and restructuring cognitive distortions about illness and recovery [1, 3]. You consider these approaches as you plan to follow Mr. Q during his hospitalization with the goals of providing support, helping him to manage distress from the existential threat of his illness and concerns about his functioning, and restoring morale along with his ability to envision a hopeful future [3].

It is important to note that the demoralization a patient is feeling may also be reflected in the experience of their medical providers. This can be the case when the medical team and patient have incongruous goals for the patient's treatment and ideas about what determines a "good" outcome. Such a mismatch in treatment goals can generate mutually frustrating attempts by both parties to feel understood and to understand the response of the other. It also highlights the importance of addressing the patient's values and goals in their treatment and maintaining open communication about the patient's wishes and concerns as they progress through treatment. The medical team may also be experiencing their own loss of morale, or an empathic, *concordant countertransference* contributing to feelings of demoralization or depression. As such, it is helpful for the medical team to be aware of demoralization in the patient and themselves and to be mindful of how it can affect their communication with the patient and the patient's participation in care.

You share with the primary team your impression that—in the setting of difficulties coping with his medical condition and catastrophic concerns about its impact on his future functioning and relationship—Mr. Q is feeling hopeless about his prognosis, as well as helpless and ambivalent about his care. In addition to following the patient supportively and assisting in linking him to outpatient psychotherapy, you guide the medical team by recommending active interventions they can make to help support Mr. Q in the hospital. You recommend that the team modify their approach to help address Mr. Q's demoralization through regular rounding and follow-up visits, maintaining an empathic stance and validating his experience, eliciting his treatment goals and addressing concerns that he expresses as he progresses in his treatment, treating or palliating any distressing physical symptoms he is experiencing including pain, and supporting the patient and his family as they transition to new roles [1]. Your impression of Mr. Q as someone who prides himself on being capable and independent—now distressed by a threat to these qualities—informs your recommendations as you help to identify strategies to encourage him to take a more active role in his care. You suggest involving the physical therapy team; collaborating with Mr. Q to set regular, reachable, and measurable functional goals that he can realistically accomplish; providing choices in the hospital when possible; and providing appropriate ongoing education about his diagnosis and treatment options. Although the team may have felt helpless and discouraged when the patient appeared depressed, providing insight into the patient's experience of his situation can restore the team's confidence in their ability to help the patient emotionally as well as medically. In doing so, both the patient and the primary medical team can begin to shift from a sense of helplessness to one of shared understanding and empowerment.

Scenario 2: Mood Disorder

As you look through Mr. Q's chart after your initial conversation with the fellow, you see that he has not required any medications for behavioral dysregulation and has no abnormal vital signs or significantly abnormal laboratory values. He received a medication the last three nights that has an indication written for "sleep", as well as a newer psychotropic that acts as both an antidepressant and a mood stabilizer that is listed as a home medication. There is a note from a social worker mentioning that he has a psychiatrist that he has seen for many years and continues to see regularly. You reconnect with the oncology fellow to get a bit more information after reviewing the chart, and he reiterates to you that Mr. Q has been disengaged from the medical team throughout his hospitalization. Other than appearing withdrawn on his mental status exam, he does not display any other symptoms of delirium and has not over the course of his hospitalization. The fellow notes that Mr. Q recently made a comment to him about the "futility" of receiving chemotherapy but that despite this he has not declined treatment. The fellow is concerned because they are not able to meaningfully discuss with him his good prognosis, his current treatment plan, or the next steps due to this unknown impairment in Mr. Q's ability to communicate with him. You wonder if the fellow feels frustrated in addition to being concerned that he is not able to share the hopeful information about Mr. Q's prognosis with him, and that if only Mr. Q could take in the information, his mood would be improved. He tells you that when he and other medical providers go into Mr. Q's room, "he barely notices we are in the room." The fellow wants to make sure they are not missing something that is contributing to his notably detached presentation such as an underlying depressed mood or hypoactive delirium.

When you enter Mr. Q's room, he is resting with his eyes closed and opens them when you introduce yourself as the psychiatric consultant. He does not say anything in response but is clearly attentive to you and making appropriate eye contact. You ask him how he has been feeling recently and he replies "okay" and then stops speaking. You attempt to initiate a conversation in multiple ways. He responds logically and coherently, but usually in only one or two word answers. You notice how hard it is to start a conversation and how his short answers create a feeling that he wants you to leave the room without his saying this overtly. You decide to try and put this into words and ask Mr. Q if he would like you to leave. He says that he does want to end the conversation since he finds it exhausting to speak to people at the moment and prefers to be alone. You see this as a potential opening and tell him that sometimes social isolation can be a symptom of depression and if he thinks that could be something he is feeling. He says yes; he knows he has been depressed for a while now and was going to ask his outpatient psychiatrist about increasing his dose of his antidepressant at their next meeting "if I make it that long." He goes on to say that he does not care what treatment he gets and that he has been going along with chemotherapy since it was easier than saying no. He does not want to talk to anyone about how he is feeling and wants to try and manage everything on his own—he hates feeling "weak" and talking about feeling depressed. If he cannot take care of himself, he does not get what the point is of "all of this." You ask him a bit more about this statement, and he says he thinks about stopping his chemotherapy and seeing what happens. He says he does not want to in reality do that, but it does feel like it is one way that he could take back control and stop being reliant on others. You empathize with how he must feel out of control while hospitalized and managing his cancer diagnosis—he agrees and says he has always been the "strong" one in his family who supports others and hates having to rely on his wife more. He does not want to be a burden on her and does not want her to have to take care of him when he leaves the hospital. You do a full safety assessment, and you do not elicit any other suicidal thoughts other than the passive suicidality he previously described.

You ask him what he understands about his diagnosis and treatment. He accurately reports the details of his surgery, but he is not sure why he needs chemotherapy and fears that it will only make him physically weaker and diminish his quality of life. You take note of how hopeless he sounds and how this is discordant with the good prognosis following chemotherapy that the fellow described. You consider what could account for this discrepancy. Is this patient cognitively distorting the information he is receiving from the medical team through a depressive and hopeless lens? Or was the medical team unable to fully discuss the details of his prognosis in a clear and thorough manner after feeling discouraged by how Mr. Q interacted with them?

You obtain permission to speak with Mr. Q's psychiatrist and give him a call. Mr. Q's psychiatrist confirms that the last time they met Mr. Q was in a depressive episode and started a new medication, the psychotropic you see in his chart, to address these depressive symptoms. He adds that Mr. Q's diagnosis is bipolar disorder and not a major depressive disorder, but he has not experienced a manic episode since his early 30s. He also confirms that Mr. Q's current psychiatric symptoms are consistent with how his prior depressive episodes presented. He is typically very engaging, is quick witted, and does not have any suicidal thoughts. During his prior mood episodes, he expressed passive suicidal thoughts but never attempted suicide. Mr. Q tends to be secretive about his bipolar disorder diagnosis and in the past has not contacted him when he was decompensating out of a desire to manage it himself and "not burden others." He thinks that Mr. Q's current hospitalization must be very difficult for him since he has previously confided in him that his worst fear is to be debilitated by an illness—whether it is bipolar disorder, cancer, or otherwise.

You approach the primary medical team and describe Mr. Q's current depressive symptoms that were present prior to his hospitalization as well as the collateral from his psychiatrist including his diagnosis of bipolar disorder. Mr. Q carries core beliefs about the meaning of being "weak" which you speculate may have led him, at least initially, to not disclose his diagnosis of bipolar disorder in order to prevent further being identified in the sick role. Ultimately, you conclude that most likely his social withdrawal, hopelessness, and minimal of interaction with the medical team can be formulated as stemming from his depressive episode as well as a psychological defense.

You describe some of the discrepancies between the information provided by the medical team and how Mr. Q processed that information. Continued patient education is important in ensuring an adequate understanding of their diagnosis and treatment recommendations as well as fostering treatment engagement [5]. Brainstorming with the medical team how to discuss his diagnosis, treatment course, and prognosis, as well as strategies to address his concerns about the meaning of his illness to him and its impact on his functioning, can be helpful. You also recommend increasing his psychotropic medication to address his depressive symptoms in coordination with his outpatient psychiatrist.

Recognizing that this patient's "disengagement" was both a symptom of depression and a defense mechanism to cope with his diagnosis of cancer helped you as the psychiatric consultant elicit his symptoms and gain the information needed to make treatment recommendations. The use of countertransference in understanding this dynamic was central to clarifying his desire to cope on his own rather than talk about his depressive symptoms. Reinforcing this patient's healthy, strong self, by continuing with chemotherapy and treatment, is one way you can use your understanding of this patient to help implement treatment recommendations.

Scenario 3: Psychological Response to a Medical Illness

The oncology fellow abruptly interrupts your initial conversation in order to answer an "emergency page." About half an hour later, he calls you back and says that the page was about Mr. Q who he just re-evaluated and who he says now needs an urgent consultation from psychiatry. The fellow tensely expresses that the patient refused to receive any additional medications through his intravenous (IV) access, including chemotherapy, and was yelling at the nurses that he needed to talk to a doctor immediately. When the fellow went to see the patient, Mr. Q was pacing, seemed on edge and very anxious, and asked for alprazolam to calm himself down. He noticed that Mr. Q was beginning to hyperventilate and then started to cry and talk rapidly about how he was going to die from cancer. The fellow quickly ordered alprazolam due to his inability to verbally de-escalate Mr. Q and his discomfort with Mr. Q's distress. The fellow has ordered alprazolam multiple times during Mr. Q's hospitalization in response to Mr. Q's request for a sleep aid or for intense anxiety similar to what the fellow just described. The fellow is not sure where the anxiety is coming from or why Mr. Q has difficulty sleeping. He wonders if Mr. Q might have an underlying benzodiazepine use disorder which leads him to exaggerate his insomnia and anxiety in order to receive alprazolam. The fellow feels conflicted about prescribing the alprazolam for that reason and also because benzodiazepines could negatively effect Mr. Q's respiratory status while he is recovering from surgery. His vital signs show a pattern of a transient reduction in respiratory rate and then subsequent increased respiratory rate a few hours later. He explains that this pattern of being paged urgently for Mr. Q's anxiety occurs multiple times a day, and he is also frequently paged to see Mr. Q for non-emergent issues such as the patient wanting further clarification or reassurance about his treatment and diagnosis. The fellow would like your help to better understand and treat Mr. Q's anxiety as well as manage the frequent time demands on him and his team.

You start to generate a differential diagnosis for Mr. Q as you walk towards his room. Is he an overtly anxious patient with poor coping skills, a disorganized and confused patient, an overmedicated patient, or a personality disordered patient? You also want to rule out any potential medical or neurologic causes to his presentation. When you arrive, Mr. Q is anxiously pacing around his room and wringing his hands. You introduce yourself to Mr. Q and explain that you were asked to see him because his medical team has noticed his increased anxiety and they wanted to see if you could help in any way. You know that he is being prescribed alprazolam by them and wanted to know if he has been finding it helpful. He replies, "Yeah, the alprazolam helps me, but that fellow doesn't seem to understand why I need it—I'm really worked up being here!" You take note of Mr. Q's feeling of being misunderstood by the fellow and wonder how that could be contributing to the dynamics between Mr. Q and the medical team. You ask Mr. Q what he wishes the fellow understood about his current situation. He tells you that it is hard for him to process that he has cancer since he was "healthy one minute, sick the next" and that he fears that he is going to die even though he knows his doctors keep telling him otherwise. As he speaks, you notice there is a dramatic flair and intense affect associated with his story and wonder if this is part of a communication strategy he unconsciously uses to maintain people's attention and presence. You find it hard to interrupt him or respond with anything other than validation of his intense feelings and find yourself looking at your watch multiple times over the course of your interview noticing how much time has passed.

Mr. Q has been perseverating over past decisions he made that may have contributed to his developing cancer and feels guilty about some of his unhealthy behaviors. He has also been ruminating about his future such as the cost of his medical care and how his diagnosis will impact his quality of life, in addition to other parts of his life not related to his diagnosis. He describes to you that he has difficulty falling asleep due to his rumination and anxiety, and when he does fall asleep, nurses constantly disturb him in order to obtain his vital signs or give him medications. He says the medications he is taking make him nauseous which makes it difficult to eat at times, but that he also usually has a reduced appetite whenever he gets stressed and anxious. He denies having any thoughts of wanting to end his life. You ask him about his symptoms of anxiety and whether he has experienced significant anxiety in the past. He tells you that he has always been a "worrier" since he was a child. He was previously in therapy and used to take alprazolam many years ago to help with his anxiety. He feels generally anxious about many things at baseline but typically is able to manage things better than he is now. He has noticed an increase in his anxiety recently after feeling more "out of control" in his life. In his first night in the hospital, he felt "panicked" so asked for alprazolam since he remembered it worked for him before. He says it is one of the few things he can do that helps him feel better.

He goes on to tell you that he has always been an independent person but that sometimes he heavily relies on his wife for reassurance and support, including making basic decisions in his life. He thinks his wife has been pulling away from him as he has become more dependent on her in the context of increasing anxiety about his diagnosis and treatment. At the same time, he also feels frustrated that she cannot understand how he feels. You reflect to yourself that this dynamic is also occurring between him and the medical team; he has felt increasingly anxious which has led to panicked interactions with them, and ultimately leads the medical team to attempt to avoid his intense anxiety by prescribing alprazolam. You can see how the medical team might feel burdened and annoyed by his frequent anxiety with no seeming cause, leading them to interpret his requests as a dependence on benzodiazepines. As a result, Mr. Q could feel alone and misunderstood, leading to an escalation in anxiety to bring the medical team's attention back to him.

From Mr. Q's perspective, you speculate that he not only looks to the alprazolam for relief from his anxiety but also as a way to feel in control when he feels out of control of his life, including his ability to receive support and reassurance. Instead of learning to tolerate his anxiety and attempt to obtain support in a more effective way, he tries to get rid of this feeling with alprazolam, creating a cycle that further reinforces his feelings of not being supported.

The stress of the hospitalization and serious illness may have contributed to Mr. Q regressing in the hospital and becoming increasingly dependent and unable to reassure himself [5]. You also hypothesize that biologically his symptoms of anxiety might be paradoxically exacerbated by his frequent alprazolam use due to its short half-life, precipitating rebound anxiety from benzodiazepine withdrawal.

After your conversation with Mr. Q, you discuss with your attending and the fellow your interactions with him. You describe Mr. Q as likely having generalized anxiety disorder (GAD) at baseline which is now exacerbated in the setting of his current medical hospitalization. You consider whether he might have dependent traits that are contributing to some of the challenging dynamics occurring. His presentation is not consistent with an adjustment disorder because his anxiety is not confined to one stressor and he has physical symptoms such as low appetite and poor sleep that is characteristic of his typical exacerbations of his generalized anxiety. You describe to them how you observed that he sometimes communicates his anxiety about his medical illness to the medical team by his behaviors and not by his words, such as asking the doctors to come to his bedside to explain things repeatedly and refusing medications through his IV for no clear reason. You acknowledge how challenging these interactions are and that this patient who desperately wants reassurance and security tends to not go about it in a way that is more adaptive, such as internalizing the reassurance from his medical team or asking directly for what he needs.

You also address the team's concern that Mr. Q may be asking for benzodiazepines due to a substance use disorder. Typical countertransference reactions that can stem from a medical team suspecting a hidden substance use disorder include feelings of resentment for ordering a medication they may not think the patient needs or feeling that the patient is using their symptoms to manipulate them. You tell the team that you too are concerned about the complexities involved in giving this patient benzodiazepines—not only because of the physical effect on the patient but also its emotional impact. You discuss with the team that short-acting alprazolam given repeatedly can cause a rebound in Mr. Q's anxiety in addition to an increase in his respiratory rate. The changes in his vital signs may reflect him becoming more anxious, receiving a dose of alprazolam, calming down, and then having rebound anxiety and physiological changes hours later. You also suggest to the team that when Mr. Q asks to be seen immediately for anxiety, it may be that he is feeling anxious about his illness or attempting to express something he needs. Validating the patient's anxiety and reminding him of coping skills he has, instead of avoiding the patient's anxiety by giving him additional alprazolam, may be a different strategy to use with him. Additionally, creating a schedule for the day where he knows when different staff will come speak to him and how long they will be speaking for will help set boundaries with Mr. Q or other patients who are requesting a lot of time from their medical team. By setting limits and expectations, patients can gain a feeling of control and predictability which can reduce anxiety. This can also help reduce feelings of anger or being overburdened that could lead to avoidance from the medical team toward the patient [5].

This is a patient with GAD who is grappling with the impact of his medical illness. As the psychiatric consultant, recognizing that a provider can respond to a patient's anxiety with avoidance or over prescribing a medication can help resolve difficult provider-patient dynamics. Interacting with this patient in a calm and consistent manner will help both the patient and team feel less anxious, allowing the team to fulfill their role in caring for the patient and for the patient to receive that care.

Appendix: Summary Table

	Problems	Strategies
• Patient symptoms and behaviors	• Mood: Dysphoria, irritability, anxiety, "inappropriate affect," overly positive, constricted range, apathetic • Behavioral disturbances: Disengagement, withdrawal, non-adherence, reluctance to talk frankly, hostility, attempts to elope, refusal of care	• Assist with diagnostic clarification and support the team in identifying and addressing underlying etiology of various presentations of depression, including delirium • Provide guidance in minimizing iatrogenic and environmental contributions to delirium • Offer easy-to-follow management recommendations, including behavioral strategies for patient redirection, re-orientation, and reassurance, and clear and thorough engagement with patient without paternalizing or patronizing • Consider pharmacologic interventions for managing mood and distressing symptoms that are interfering with safety or care. May also aid in directing team's approach to sensorium of patient and reducing iatrogenic negative aspects of hospital setting and reducing polypharmacy
• Provider-patient dynamics	• Provider with countertransference feelings including projecting one's own feelings about the patient's situation onto the patient (e.g., "He's so young, it's so sad") • Provider discomfort with psychological content of patient, unwilling to explore emotional impact of illness (e.g., "He must be depressed, call psych") • Patient feeling unsupported by providers leading to withdrawal or despair. Patients can experience the lack of emotional connectedness from their providers as abandonment and cause them to act out in various ways, as well as influence the reaction in turn that comes from the provider	• Validate the experience of the provider, talking through their emotional response to the patient and their role in caring for the patient. Empathize with their difficult role in caring for patient, also to model for the team a way of engaging the patient • Provide a clear diagnosis and psychoeducation, help the team recognize variable presentations of adjusting to an illness, and make sense of frustrating, confusing, or unusual behaviors from patients • Outline active interventions to be made to help the patient and re-empower the team, through reengaging patient, educating patient, and sharing an honest "human" stance versus a solely "doctor" stance to illness with the patient

• Inter-provider and provider-family dynamics	• Team attributes symptoms to an underlying psychiatric disorder (e.g., depression, psychotic disorder), leading to sense of being unable to help, loss of "ownership" of treatment, a drive to transfer patient, or limiting further medical management in lieu of alternative care • Family distressed about medical and physical condition of patient and projecting their own discomfort/despair onto patient or providers • Family distressed about acute cognitive and behavioral changes, or medical and physical interventions being used for management, and reflect their anger or despair to the providers who may feel it more intensely as coming from both the patient and family and possibly unconsciously from themselves	• Provide a clear presentation and interpretation of symptoms and observed behaviors, as psychoeducation for the primary team and family. May remark explicitly if there are no primary psychiatric comorbidities or contributions to current presentation, or more likely the nuances attributed to variable factors of the situation • Assist in guiding and expanding primary team's thinking about the patient's role in family and impact on family trying to understand the changing image of their family member. Educate family about depression, stress reactions, conditions like delirium that can happen when someone is in the hospital, and expectations around recovery (if known), and explain empathically that efforts are made to maintain patient's safety • Support family in their distress and provide receptive space for both providers and family to feel their feelings and discuss the impact of illness, perhaps in a family meeting or by guiding the medical providers on how to discuss with family
• Patient-provider barriers	• Cognitive and affective impairment associated with depression, illness, or neurocognitive disorder limiting patient's understanding in communications with providers and what can or should be done, or issues with capacity • Patient may not want to disclose sensitive information if they feel vulnerable with the team or ashamed or other feelings they may want to avoid	• Provide cognitively impaired patients with clear, consistent and concrete explanations. Identify and elicit support from family or next of kin. If changes in treatment need to happen, explain thoroughly and have patient and/or family repeat back their understanding • Providers should approach perceived nonadherence with open non-aggressive confrontation, and consider emotional impact of illness on patient, asking explicitly about their observations and giving patient ample time to respond, ask questions, discuss concerns, and feel heard

(continued)

	Problems	Strategies
• Hospital system barriers	• Patient safety can become an obtuse non-meaningful goal that leads to lack of understanding and frustration for patient and provider, and hospital administration oversight that puts pressure on providers unnecessarily, can create a tense environment • Patient's challenges in managing their illness lead to recurrent hospitalizations and high healthcare utilization	• Patient safety should be a joint collaboration with all those involved with clear goals and directives. Consider additional provider and staff education around psychoeducation and common hospital occurrences, behavioral management and redirection, standing pharmacologic interventions and creative changes in environment to make use of least restrictive means necessary for safety • Psychoeducation for family and patient and providing adequate outpatient support via appointments, easy access to information, and contingency planning can help patient feel more empowered, less likely to utilize a higher resource when not necessary, and avoid waiting until a condition is worsening before seeking care

References

1. Sansone RA, Sansone LA. Demoralization in patients with medical illness. Psychiatry (Edgemont). 2010;7(8):42–5. https://www.ncbi.nlm.nih.gov/pmc/articles/PMC2945856/.
2. Clarke DM, Kissane DW. Demoralization: its phenomenology and importance. Aust N Z J Psychiatry. 2002;36(6):733–42. https://doi.org/10.1046/j.1440-1614.2002.01086.x.
3. Caruso R, Giuliananni M, Riba MB, Sabato S, Grassi L. Depressive spectrum disorders in cancer: diagnostic issues and intervention. A critical review. Curr Psychiatry Rep. 2017;19(6):33. https://doi.org/10.1007/s11920-017-0785-7.
4. O'Keeffe N, Ranjith G. Depression, demoralisation or adjustment disorder? Understanding emotional distress in the severely medically ill. Clin Med (Lond). 2007;7(5):478–81. https://doi.org/10.7861/clinmedicine.7-5-478.
5. Green SA. Psychotherapeutic principles and techniques: principles of medical psychotherapy. In: Barry SF, Donna BG, editors. Psychiatric care of the medical patient. 3rd ed. Oxford: Oxford University Press; 2015. p. 191–204.

Major Neurocognitive Disorder

13

Melanie Bilbul and Jennifer Finkel

The pager reads: "The patient can't engage with the team—can you help us?"

Your first task in clarifying the primary team's question is understanding what is meant by "can't engage with the team." Having a more clear understanding of what the team means by "engage" and what factors make "engagement" difficult is essential to figuring out how to best help the team. Are there functional impairments the patient has demonstrated prior to and during their hospitalization? Additional questions can involve gathering specific information from the patient's history as well as through what the patient's interactions have been like thus far with the team. Is there a lack of engagement or inappropriate engagement? A lack of engagement could be reflected by a patient not answering questions, not taking medications or a reduced level of arousal due to various etiologies. Examples of inappropriate engagement include disinhibition or impulsivity, such as when a patient exhibits physical aggression towards clinical staff. A lack of engage-

M. Bilbul (✉)
Department of Psychiatry and Addictology, University of Montreal, Montreal, QC, Canada
e-mail: melanie.bilbul.med@ssss.gouv.qc.ca

J. Finkel
Department of Psychiatry, Icahn School of Medicine at Mount Sinai, New York, NY, USA

A. Gorun et al. (eds.), *The Psychiatric Consult*,
https://doi.org/10.1007/978-3-031-26837-3_13

ment and inappropriate engagement can both be found in patients experiencing major neurocognitive disorders and other disorders. Questions about onset and time course can be useful for creating and sorting through differential diagnoses.

Neurocognitive disorders can have slow, insidious onsets or can be rapidly progressive. They can result in cognitive and physical limitations, as well as psychiatric symptomatology. The differential diagnosis for cognitive issues is broad and can include delirium, depressive disorders, psychotic disorders, and substance use disorders. Keeping your differential diagnosis in mind will be helpful in targeting your questions and determining the appropriate diagnosis and treatment.

Beyond asking for help in the management of the patient, the team may also be asking *why* the patient is unable to engage with the team. They may be hoping that there is a psychiatric diagnosis or component to the patient's behavior that the psychiatric consultant can magically change. Carefully assessing for both psychiatric and non-psychiatric contributions to the patient's presentation will help the team determine the appropriate intervention. At times, the role of the psychiatric consultant is to communicate that there is *not* a psychiatric origin to the patent's behavior. Guiding the team to utilize the appropriate clinicians and other specialties or further workup would then be the next recommendation.

Clinical Scenario

After receiving the page, you start by reviewing the chart prior to speaking to the primary team requesting the consult. You learn that Mr. X is an 84-year-old retired carpenter who has lived alone since his wife died 1 year ago. He has one married adult daughter and two grandchildren. He has a medical history of hypertension, dyslipidemia, type 2 diabetes mellitus, and peripheral vascular disease. His only listed psychiatric and neurologic history is a diagnosis of major neurocognitive disorder made by his primary care provider 2 years ago. He has a family history of Alzheimer's disease, which his mother was diagnosed with in her 80s. He has a 50 pack-year smoking history and quit 15 years ago. He denies any substance use. Mr. X presented to the emergency room with unilateral right lower extremity edema. Within a few hours of presentation, he developed a fever and began to have redness in his leg, and his edema and pain worsened. He was ultimately diagnosed with necrotizing fasciitis and hospitalized. The notes from the surgical team indicate that they are recommending a below the knee amputation (BKA) to control the infection.

Scenario 1: Capacity Assessment

You call back the vascular surgery resident to begin to clarify the team's question. She tells you that Mr. X was previously agreeing to their treatment recommendations until they recommended a BKA, which he has adamantly refused. The resident is worried that the patient does not have decision-making capacity because of his documented neurocognitive disorder and would like you to assess his capacity to refuse the amputation.

As you hear more about the nature of the team's request for a decision-making capacity assessment and ask follow-up questions, it is important that you keep in mind a conceptual overview that includes the following: what is decision-making capacity, how is it assessed, and in what ways is its assessment relevant to the current problem that the team and patient are having.

What Is Decision-Making Capacity?

Decision-making capacity is a person's ability to choose a course of action related to their body or health and assumes that the person has appropriate information to make that choice. Decision-making capacity assessments are specific to the decision that needs to be made and to the current moment in time. It is appropriate, for example, to assess decision-making capacity to refuse vital signs, bloodwork, medications, procedures, or aspects of the discharge plan, if these issues are actively being negotiated between the patient and the treatment team. It would not be appropriate to assess decision-making capacity about a future decision, or about global decision-making. Determination of global abilities in a few distinct areas, such as the ability to make decisions related to one's body or related to one's finances (otherwise known as competency), will sometimes be required in the case of an individual with a significant neurocognitive or psychiatric issue. However, such determinations are made by the court system—not by a clinician in the hospital—and are not relevant to the acute needs of an often urgent nature that arise during a hospital stay. It may be relevant if the patient has already been deemed to not be competent in one of these areas and documentation of this has been confirmed.

How Is Decision-Making Capacity Assessed?

Most clinicians use criteria described by Paul Appelbaum: can the patient communicate a consistent choice regarding treatment preference; can the patient demonstrate understanding of the relevant information about the illness and proposed treatment(s); does the patient appear to rationally manipulate the information relevant to the situation; and does the patient demonstrate appreciation of the situation and the consequences of the choice(s) they are making [1]. Although any physician can assess for capacity, often psychiatry is involved for more nuanced, complex cases, where there are questions about how the mental status or psychiatric issues are affecting the decision-making process. In some cases, a hospital's medical ethics team may be consulted—for example, if there are significant concerns that the patient's stated choice puts them in imminent danger, when a determination that the patient does not have decision-making capacity may involve substantially overriding the patient's autonomy, or in other complicated situations with significant implications on the health and well-being of the patient, and where another perspective would be helpful. A representative of the hospital administration is often helpful or necessary in cases where the patient is not demonstrating decision-making capacity and does not have a designated surrogate decision-maker.

In addition to the criteria outline by Applebaum [1], decision-making capacity assessments may also be subject to a sliding scale, which stipulates that a more stringent standard of capacity should be applied to situations where the patient's decision embodies a higher risk [2, 3]. According to Drane [3], the potential risk and accorded stringency of decision-making capacity can be divided into three tiers. In the first scenario, the least rigorous criteria for decision-making capacity are applied in cases where the proposed treatment is effective and carries minimal risk and there are few or no alternatives. Here, the patient is only required to be "aware of what is going on," and their assent alone is the rational expectation for decision-making capacity. A second standard of decision-making capacity is applied where the illness is more chronic (rather than acute), or if the treatment carries a higher risk or less definite benefit, or if there are alternatives to treatment. In this situation, the patient must also exhibit an understanding of the proposed treatment, the risk, benefits, and alternatives to the treatment. The third and most stringent standard of decision-making capacity is applied in dangerous clinical situations where an effective and life-saving treatment is available, and refusal of treatment will likely result in severe morbidity or death. In this scenario, patients must meet all the criteria outlined by Appelbaum [1].

How Will the Decision-Making Capacity Assessment Impact Clinical Care?

There are some cases where a team will request a decision-making capacity determination but where it is evident that it is not relevant or where its determination may not specifically solve the problem at hand. For example, decision-making capacity to refuse oral medications for a chronic medical condition can technically be assessed (i.e., refusal to accept this medication today), but does not have a clear value when it comes to a condition that requires daily medication taking over months and years, such as in the management of HIV disease. It would be useful to assess decision-making capacity for a patient actively refusing insulin with a blood sugar of 800 and actively at risk of developing diabetic ketoacidosis, but assessing decision-making capacity to refuse an oral hypoglycemic medication in a patient with mild type 2 diabetes who has high, but not imminently life-threatening, blood sugar levels, and where the risk is actually related to their long-term adherence with the treatment is not a clearly helpful question to answer. One part of the consultant's job prior to doing a capacity assessment is to understand whether making a capacity determination is the most relevant question to providing appropriate care for the patient, or whether answering a different question will be more useful. For example, understanding what barriers exist that are leading to the patient's nonadherence, and helping to improve them, may be a more useful question. Another important part is considering what happens after the psychiatric consultant determines the patient's decision-making capacity. For example, if the patient is deemed to not demonstrate decision-making capacity, are there any interventions that can restore it, such as treating physical or psychiatric factors affecting the patient's decision-making. If there is no way to restore it, is there a way of reframing the options such that the patient can assent to the most important recommendations from the team? This would mean the patient agrees to a treatment without having decision-making capacity. Is there some aspect of the interaction between the patient and provider that the psychiatric consultant can modify so they can have a more effective conversation?

With this framework in mind, you continue to gather information from the vascular surgery resident. The resident is concerned that without an amputation Mr. X. may become septic and have a high risk of mortality. She also explains to you the risks of morbidity and mortality associated with the surgery itself, including bleeding, the spread of the infection despite surgery, and the risks of anesthesia. You clarify the expected course of recovery for a man of Mr. X's age and general health from the surgery and ask if there are any alternatives to the surgery. The resident responds that at this point in time, there is none. Based on the clinical information you have gathered, you conclude that you will need to use a higher stringency for assessing decision-making capacity according to the sliding scale principle, given that it is an acute, life-threatening situation where an effective treatment (i.e., amputation) is available, and refusal of treatment will likely result in sepsis and death. This stringency must be balanced by taking into account the patient's autonomy, including the right to refuse potentially lifesaving proposed treatments, a cornerstone of medical ethics [4]. When a patient is refusing a lifesaving treatment, this can result in a particularly strong countertransference of wanting to save the patient from death. This may cause the psychiatrist to fall into a "convincer role" for the patient, rather than performing an objective assessment of their capacity. It is important for the psychiatrist to not get overly pulled into medical aspects of the case and to not let the fact that the patient's doctors feel the patient is making the "wrong" decision influence their assessment.

Now that you understand more about the treatment recommendation, your focus turns to understanding what factors may be influencing the patient's decision-making. You ask the resident to clarify what exactly the patient said when he decided to not have the surgery. She answers, "I'm not sure. He kept saying that there 'must be some mistake' and 'no, I don't want to do that' and wouldn't elaborate any further." You then ask the vascular surgical resident how the patient has been behaving in his interactions with the team. More specifically, which forms of medical care has the patient agreed to? Is refusing? Has he seemed confused or experienced a change in his level of consciousness or behavior over the course of the hospitalization? The resident replies that Mr. X has been very cooperative with their recommendations up until this point, taking all of his medications and accepting intravenous antibiotics. He has not missed any doses. He has been pleasant with the staff. The resident expresses she was surprised when Mr. X refused their recommendation for surgery, given his consent to all other forms of treatment that had been initiated. He has not appeared confused or had a change in mental status that she has noticed. The resident emphasizes that she needs your help to figure out what to do because the operating room needs to be booked quickly. After reviewing his vital signs and bloodwork, you note the only abnormality is an elevated white blood cell count.

Following a review of the chart and discussion with the primary team, you are now ready to see the patient. In the hospital, the primary team, and not the patient, may be requesting a psychiatric consult. The primary team should then always inform the patient of a plan for a psychiatric consultation since the patient may have preconceived notions and biases about psychiatry that the primary team can address, not understand their role in their treatment, or refuse the consultation altogether. These may be based on prior experiences with mental healthcare providers, their cultural background, or other factors. There may also be general beliefs about doctors and the healthcare system, including the need to be overly deferential or feelings of suspiciousness. Therefore, it is crucial that the primary team tell the patient the reason for the consult and allow the patient space to ask questions. It can also at times be beneficial for the primary team to join the psychiatrist for their initial meeting with the patient to facilitate communication and have an effective consult.

When you enter Mr. X's room, you notice he is calmly lying in bed eating lunch. You introduce yourself to Mr. X and the reason his surgical team requested a consultation. Mr. X is visibly annoyed. He replies, "Why are they sending a psychiatrist? I'm not crazy!" You apologize that he wasn't informed that you'd be meeting with him and focus on building rapport, which allows the interview to continue. He tells you that he is in shock that he needs an amputation since his foot looked fine to him up until he got to the hospital and that he wishes his wife was still alive to help him make medical decisions. You then begin to ask questions relevant to the capacity assessment while thinking of the four criteria outlined by Applebaum [1]. You ask Mr. X what he understands about his diagnosis and the treatment recommendations of his team. He explains that he knows he has an infection that is spreading quickly. You ask him what the doctors have suggested as treatment and whether he knows the risks and benefits of the proposed treatments. He says, "They want to cut off my leg… I know if they don't do it, I might die. If I do it, I might bleed a lot. They also said something about the anesthesia that I can't remember." When asked about any alternatives to having surgery, he answers, "There aren't any." You then ask him what he thinks should be the next step in his treatment, and to your surprise he says he thinks he should get the surgery. You point out that to the surgical team he said he did not want to get the surgery but now would like to go ahead with the surgery—what made him change his mind? He replies, "I've always been a fighter. I want to live." You notice yourself feeling confused, and you try asking again since he has not answered the question of why he changed his mind. He says that he does not remember ever refusing to get an amputation and cannot think of any reasons why he would have refused it since it would save his life. You wonder if this inconsistency may be due to a cognitive impairment, and you realize you did not conduct a formal mental status exam yet. The resident's assessment that there was no confusion or mental status exam changes present may have influenced you to not think that one was necessary for this patient. When you conduct your mental status exam you discover that both his orientation and his attention are impaired.

Capacity assessments are structured and direct. You determined that Mr. X appreciates the situation and relevant information (risk and benefits of the surgery as well as not pursuing surgery); however, he does not express a choice clearly and cannot provide a consistent and logical reply. This shows he has difficulty manipulating information rationally. At this point, you have determined that the patient lacks capacity to participate in an informed care discussion regarding the BKA. He was only able to meet two of the four of Appelbaum's criteria: appreciating the situation and relevant information.

You are concerned this patient may be delirious on top of his previously diagnosed neurocognitive disorder. With Mr. X's permission, you call his daughter to assess whether the patient's mental status exam is worse than his baseline, as well as to verify the patient's psychiatric history and any risk factors relevant to ensuring his safety. When you speak to her on the phone, she tells you she visited Mr. X this morning and was upset with how quickly his memory seemed to have decline. She says that he was "not making any sense" and thought that his wife was still alive. He had never thought she was still alive prior to this hospitalization, and despite his cognitive deficits, she had always been able to have coherent and full conversations with him. She denies her father having any history of self-injury, suicidal thoughts, violence, agitation, or wandering.

You call the resident back to inform her of your determination that the patient is not demonstrating decision-making capacity to consent to surgery. You explain that a delirium superimposed on his underlying neurocognitive disorder is high on your differential based on your mental status exam and from the collateral from his daughter, as well as the multiple risk factors he has for delirium including his recent infection and older age. It would be best to turn to his healthcare proxy at this point to make the clinical decision based on the proxy's best effort to make a choice consistent with the patient's values. It will be the primary team's responsibility to engage the daughter in the discussion regarding the surgery and goals of care following your capacity assessment. Of note, the presence of a cognitive impairment does not necessarily preclude someone from having capacity to make medical decisions. All adults are typically presumed to have capacity until it is determined otherwise. A critical point in educating primary teams about capacity issues in their patients is that decision-making capacity is specific, can change over time, and cannot be generalized to other points in time or to other decisions.

Capacity assessments can provoke strong countertransference reactions and interpersonal dilemmas for clinicians. For example, after deciding that someone lacks decision-making capacity, the psychiatric consultant can be overwhelmed by the thought that they are forcing someone to receive a treatment against their will and overriding their autonomy. However, it is important to keep in mind that the psychiatrist is only determining a patient's capacity, and it is ultimately up to the primary team to make appropriate treatment recommendations and then for a surrogate or a judge to ultimately make the final decision. In some cases, family members can help provide information about what the person would have wanted prior to losing their capacity, which can be helpful in relieving feelings of guilt or worry about harming a patient. Another common countertransference dilemma occurs in cases where the person has capacity, but the psychiatrist disagrees with the decision the patient is making. If a person has capacity, their choice should be respected, no matter how irrational it may seem, or harmful it may be. It is important for the psychiatrist to maintain neutrality, notice any strong feelings, and not let these affect the assessment.

Clinical Scenario

Mr. X is a 74-year-old man who is a widower and lives alone since his wife died a year ago. He is a retired lawyer, with no children, and is an active volunteer within his community. He has a past medical history of hypertension and dyslipidemia and a suspected transient ischemic attack 3 years ago and is an active smoker. His primary care doctor diagnosed him with a major neurocognitive disorder. He was admitted to the hospital for a left total hip arthroplasty, after he tripped at home and fell. The primary team calls you a week after his surgery because Mr. X has been "agitated" for the past few days. This includes him shouting in the middle of the night, cursing at staff members, being combative with nurses, and attempting to get out of bed without assistance which resulted in an additional fall during his hospitalization. When you speak to the resident he tells you, "Mr. X requires a lot of time and attention from our nursing staff, and at this point they are not sure they can handle him anymore. The cursing and combativeness have been getting worst since he was first admitted." He also tells you that Mr. X's behavior has started to interfere with his ability to receive physical therapy. Mr. X is awaiting placement in a subacute rehabilitation facility, and the resident is concerned that his behavioral disturbances will delay placement.

Scenario 2: Agitation

When you review the chart, you note that Mr. X received two doses of a benzodiazepine yesterday and three times today. He has intermittently required soft, two-point restraints after being combative with staff. You also see notes that indicate that although his infection is cleared, he intermittently refuses to participate in physical therapy. He has no known history of substance use per the chart, and he does not exhibit any symptoms of alcohol withdrawal including stable vital signs the last 2 days. He has no known history of a psychiatric disorder, suicide attempts, or violence documented as well. Importantly, you keep in mind that both delirium and neurocognitive disorder can present with mood and psychotic symptoms. This can be an important teaching point for the primary team, as it is not uncommon for physicians not trained in psychiatry to suspect a primary psychiatric issue when presented with mood or psychotic symptoms, rather than a medical origin. You note head imaging done 1 year ago indicating loss of parenchymal volume and chronic microvascular changes and a recent head cat-scan after his fall that showed no acute changes. Additionally, there are Mini-Mental Status Exam (MMSE) [5] scores that declined over the course of the hospitalization from 23 to 18, increasing your suspicion of a superimposed delirium on his underlying major neurocognitive disorder.

Prior to seeing Mr. X, you speak with his nurse. In all consultations—and particularly for patients with neurocognitive disorders and behavioral disturbances where a patient's memory or ability to provide recent history may be affected—nurses and other direct caregivers can provide invaluable insight into the patient's behaviors, behavioral antecedents and patterns, and responses to staff interventions. The nurse tells you that Mr. X is mostly accepting of care but becomes more confused in the evenings and will begin to yell out for his wife or ask to go home. The nurse reports that Mr. X has been repeatedly trying to get out of bed without assistance, yells out purposelessly, and requires constant reassurance and redirection overnight. He sometimes yells or becomes combative when the overnight staff try to take his vital signs or do bloodwork. The nurse notes that sometimes verbal redirection is ineffective, and the team has attempted to give benzodiazepines to reduce his agitation. Her staff feels overwhelmed and frequently pages the primary team in desperation for additional benzodiazepines when they feel things are getting out control. Soft restraints were sometimes necessary to keep staff safe since he is "such a violent person" and can't "just leave everyone alone." You take note that the nurse is interpreting the patient's behavior as volitional and as part of his personality. You also notice how the feelings of the staff are influencing the requests for pharmacologic management of the patient.

When you enter Mr. X's room, you notice he is alert, has an uneaten tray of food next to him, and appears somewhat anxious. You introduce yourself as a member of the psychiatry team. As you begin to talk to him, you immediately notice that he is grossly disorganized and inattentive. Your MMSE is consistent with the previously documented moderate impairment, confirming that his mental status has deteriorated over the course of the hospitalization. When you screen for the presence of delusions and other psychotic symptoms, he says that he does not understand why he is here and why he cannot go home and expresses some mild paranoia about the nurses and other staff. He starts to get increasingly anxious and afraid and starts to try to take off his covers to get out of bed. You start to feel panicked—what if he gets out of bed and injures himself–and attempt to re-direct him by explaining why he is in the hospital and that maybe he should eat the uneaten dinner that is by his bedside. He luckily responds to your verbal de-escalation, but you can see how quickly Mr. X escalates and why the nurses and staff feel anxious to give him medication to stay in bed to control him.

You decide to meet with the resident and nurse together to provide education and make recommendations to help manage his behavior. You describe the pattern that leads to escalation of Mr. X's behavior—namely how his confusion and mild paranoia leads him to engage in potential unsafe behaviors, leading to administration of benzodiazepines, which likely contributed even more to his confusion and delirium. Medications such as benzodiazepines, antihistamines, and anticholinergics can worsen delirium in the elderly, so you instead recommend use of an antipsychotic such as haloperidol if medication management is needed. In order to try to reduce the need of pharmacological management and physical restraints, you remind the resident and nurse of the evidence base behind behavioral interventions such as having a patient care attendant be at his bedside to re-orient him and placing familiar objects in his room [6]. You recommend that any vital signs or blood draws that are not necessary to be reduced and to attempt to not have his overnight sleep be disrupted. You also empathize with their desire to control Mr. X—he is potentially putting himself and the staff in danger, but that the current administration of benzodiazepines will likely only prolong his course in the hospital rather than help him be discharged.

Agitation is a common consult in consultation-liaison psychiatry. It is important to discern the specific behavior that is being described as agitation and to consider the cause of the behavior in the context of your leading diagnosis. Medications and restraints to manage agitation should only be used in cases when a patient is at an imminent risk of harming themselves or others, or in severe distress. A clear and step-wise behavioral and pharmacologic plan can be developed with the primary team to manage staff member's frustration and anxiety about a patient and to reduce the risk of under or over medicating a patient.

Patient-team dynamics can also influence the perception of the patient's behavior. For example, episodic outbursts may be inaccurately viewed as a patient being willfully disruptive, when they are the result of a medical or neurologic cause. The staff may also experience anxiety and fear for their own safety when providing care for agitated patients, which can affect their decision-making. Team members who are feeling overwhelmed or deskilled in managing such behaviors may react with unintentional overreliance on pharmacologic interventions, or with the use of unnecessary physical restraints—each of which carries increased risk for iatrogenic harm and must be used judiciously when behavioral and environmental interventions are insufficient for maintaining safety. Keep an eye out for these potential dynamics when called about agitation, and use the opportunity to educate the team about the cause of agitation and how to safely manage it.

Clinical Scenario

Mr. X is an 81-year-old man who is single, has an adult son, and lives alone. He is a retired taxi driver. He has a past medical history of colon cancer treated with a bowel resection 10 years ago, type 2 diabetes, major neurocognitive disorder, and hypertension.

His family doctor suggested he present to the emergency room after experiencing several months of poor nutrition and weight loss. He was admitted to a geriatrics inpatient unit and diagnosed with failure to thrive.

Scenario 3: Failure to Thrive

You call the geriatrics fellow back after receiving the page. He tells you that he is concerned that Mr. X spends most of the day with his eyes closed, lying in bed, and not responding to any questions from staff or primary team. His nurse said he sometimes will suddenly shout loudly, but won't respond to any questions when asked about it. His mental status is consistent throughout the day and night with no waxing or waning symptoms. The fellow thinks Mr. X's symptoms of social withdrawal, lack of appetite, and sleep disturbance, in addition to not participating in physical therapy, are due to depression. He tells you they have completed their medical workup with no significant findings that could explain his behavior or weight loss. The fellow seems concerned and preoccupied with Mr. X, telling you it pains him to watch him slowly withdraw from the world and that he knows if it was his father he would want to do everything he could to help him. His own father suffered with depression and never got it treated. You take note of the fellow's association to his own father and wonder to yourself if that could be influencing the consult question. He asks you to assess whether a psychiatric medication might help his depression and perhaps reverse some of the progressive functional decline that has occurred.

You review the chart and confirm that his vital signs and laboratory results ordered thus far have been overall within normal limits with the exception of a low albumin, which indicates malnutrition. The chart, however, does not contain as much information as you expected regarding the patient, and you notice that there is an incomplete workup of this patient's weight loss. You note that the patient has had a declining MMSE score, most recently in the past few months between 12 and 8. You suspect some inter-administrator variability; nevertheless, both scores indicate that the patient has had long-standing, increasingly severe cognitive deficits. There is no history of a psychiatric illness in the chart.

You start to think about your differential for this patient. This includes a major depressive disorder, end-stage symptoms of neurocognitive disorder, hypoactive delirium, recent stroke with residual symptoms of apathy, and medical causes contributing to depression or apathy. You note that there is further medical workup that has not been completed by the primary team, including ruling out endocrine contributions such as thyroid abnormalities or a pituitary mass or screening for cancer.

It is not uncommon for end-stage neurocognitive disorders to present as "depressive disorders" due to the noted apathy, social withdrawal, poor oral intake, disrupted sleep, irritability, and unpredictable behavior. Endicott's criteria, which focus more on the psychological symptoms rather than the physical or somatic symptoms of depressive disorders, can be used to clarify your diagnosis [7]. These include symptoms such as increased tearfulness or depressed appearance and pessimism. Neither of these symptoms are present in this patient based on the chart review.

When you go see the patient, he appears frail and is lying in bed. He does not open his eyes when you speak to him and does not follow 1-step commands. You press his nailbed, an uncomfortable action, but necessary to assess whether he responds to painful stimuli or is comatose. The patient responds to pain by shifting, opening his eyes, and then closing them back again. You are unable to re-engage him. You try repeating his name and he suddenly shouts "No! I want to leave!" You stop talking and he goes back to sleep. At this point, you have gathered enough data about the patient's mental status exam and decide to speak to a collateral source in order to get more information.

You call the patient's son to gather some more information about his symptoms and their time course. He explains that his father has had declining cognition for many years and had help with bathing, dressing, cooking, and cleaning and managing his finances and medications for the past 2 years. However, he used to spontaneously eat and participate in conversation which now over the past few months has progressively declined. He is also concerned that he is sleeping all the time. He does not think he is depressed; he has never suffered from any psychiatric illness. There is no history of substance use, violence, self-injury, or suicide. His father was very self-motivated, engaged, and productive prior to the onset of his neurocognitive disorder.

Based on your chart review, interview of the patient, and collateral from the son, you determine that the patient's presentation is most likely related to his late-stage neurocognitive disorder rather than a depression. You also place hypoactive delirium low on your differential given the slow and progressive symptom onset and lack of waxing and waning symptoms. However, given the significant change in eating and social interaction, it is still important to do a full medical workup to identify any potentially treatable causes of these changes. Often patients at this stage are unable to meaningful engage with others and sleep most of the time with bouts of dysregulated behavior.

You call the fellow to discuss your findings and recommendations, and he agrees that he can order the additional tests you recommended. You discuss with him how this will be important to determine the cause of his admission and how a psychiatric diagnosis, especially in someone with no history of psychiatric illness, is a diagnosis of exclusion. You also tell him that at this point he should move forward with goals of care discussions and determine what his prognosis is, including whether hospice is indicated. He seems disappointed by this and asks you "is there really nothing else we can do?" You empathize with the fellow's feeling of helplessness and re-frame the goals of care discussion as an active intervention to best take care of the patient.

Providers may have strong feelings regarding patients with neurocognitive disorders, who are often debilitated and with few options for treatment. They may find themselves uncharacteristically detached and avoidant when interacting with a patient, or alternatively have an overly protective and potentially parental approach, including a desire to do "everything" beyond what is expected or reasonable. It is also important to be aware that emotional experiences that occur while caring for vulnerable elderly patients may be influenced by a myriad of past personal experiences with either ailing loved ones or prior patients. In this scenario, the fellow may have been over identifying Mr. X with his own father, influencing his clinical decision-making. Additionally, people working in a helping role (e.g., doctors, social workers, nurses) may have a strong motivation to be experienced as *helpful* by patients and their families, which can lead to uncomfortable feelings of ineffectiveness and helplessness when there are few treatment options. As psychiatric consultants, it can be helpful to assist primary teams to recognize these emotions by providing validation all the while discussing realistic options and limitations to care [8]. These steps can help teams persevere in the medical workup, remain objective in their approach, and feel supported overall.

In this scenario, recognizing and addressing the fellow's feelings of helplessness regarding the patient can be key in ultimately having the team mobilize a necessary workup and conversation with the family. Being mindful of the psychology of the patient, his family, members of the primary team, and ourselves ultimately help to ensure an objective assessment of the patient, their needs, and complex circumstances.

Appendix: Summary Table

	Problems	Strategies
• *Patient symptoms and behaviors*	• Neurocognitive disorders increase risk for delirium	• Frequent orientation, visual and hearing aids, regulate sleep-wake cycle. Approach in a holistic way and consult social work, occupational therapy, and other resources to assist patient • Involve patient's family when appropriate • Medication for any behavior that involves acute dangerousness to self or others, weighing risks and benefits of these medications
• *Provider-patient dynamics*	• May provoke feelings of provider ineffectiveness and hopelessness • May elicit provider rescue fantasies	• Empower team through psychoeducation, supporting their strengths and the positive work they have done and can do, empathize, and "sit with the feelings" of helplessness or frustration, provide concrete and active interventions that the team can make to facilitate care, be available for questions and guidance • Self-reflect and maintain awareness of our own countertransference (towards patient and team), seek supervision, and communicate with mentors to understand our response and maintain objectivity
• *Patient-provider barriers*	• Memory deficits may affect ability to remember providers, understand and recall medical issues, recommendations, treatments	• Use frequent memory aids (e.g., visual cues, calendars, written materials) • Provide time for reorienting the patient to provider role in patient care and to medical and treatment situation • Involve family or healthcare proxy to support and advocate for the patient, assist patient and team with guiding treatment and decision-making when appropriate

(continued)

	Problems	Strategies
• *Hospital system barriers*	• Hospital cannot always accommodate patients who are "slow" to recover, have irreversible deficits as in neurodegenerative conditions • Increased length of stay and difficulty transitions to long-term care as a result of behavioral disturbances • Limited options for disposition and limited supportive services for families of people with neurocognitive disorders	• Encourage team to utilize available hospital-based resources, determine level of care needed by patient • Recommend or initiate collaborative team meetings and family meetings, which may include social work, nursing and medical staff in effort to formulate safe disposition plan, identify and troubleshoot disposition difficulties • Utilize behavioral, environmental, and hospital-based resources to address behavioral difficulties and facilitate safe disposition • Weigh risk/benefit of discharging patient prior to full resolution of symptoms, reassure family, and provide tools and resources for family in case behavior escalates • Enlist help from community resources, refer early, maintain a multidisciplinary approach throughout

References

1. Appelbaum P. Assessment of patients' competence to consent to treatment. N Engl J Med. 2007;357(18):1834–40.
2. Lim T, Marin D. The assessment of decisional capacity. Neurol Clin. 2011;29(1):115–26.
3. Drane J. Competency to give an informed consent: a model for making clinical assessments. JAMA. 1984;25(7):925–7.
4. Chaet D. AMA Code of Medical Ethics' opinions on patient decision-making capacity and competence and surrogate decision making. AMA J Ethics. 2017;19(7):675–7.
5. Folstein M, Robins L, Helzer J. The mini-mental state examination. Arch Gen Psychiatry. 2017;40(7):812.
6. Cerejeira J, Lagarto L, Mukaetova-Ladinska E. Behavioral and psychological symptoms of dementia. Front Neurol. 2012;3:73. https://doi.org/10.3389/fneur.2012.00073.

7. Saracino RM, Rosenfeld B, Nelson C. Towards a new conceptualization of depression in older adult cancer patients: a review of the literature. Aging Ment Health. 2016;20(12):1230–42.
8. Morgan AC. Practical geriatrics: psychodynamic psychotherapy with older adults. Psychiatr Serv. 2003;54(12):1592–4.

Further Reading

Genevay B, Katz RS. Countertransference and older clients. Newbury Park: SAGE; 1990.

McKeith IG, Boeve BF, Dickson DW. Diagnosis and management of dementia with Lewy bodies: fourth consensus report of the DLB Consortium. Neurology. 2017;89(1):88–100. https://doi.org/10.1212/WNL.0000000000004058.

Index

A. Gorun et al. (eds.), *The Psychiatric Consult*, https://doi.org/10.1007/978-3-031-26837-3